# PANACEA
## IN MY VEINS


Reading furnishes the mind only with materials of knowledge;
it is thinking that makes what we read ours.

~John Locke

# PANACEA
## IN MY VEINS

Stem Cell Facts and Fiction

FARRUKH HAMID, MD. MSc. MBA

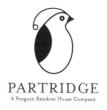

PARTRIDGE
A Penguin Random House Company

**To order additional copies of this book, contact**
Toll Free 800 101 2657 (Singapore)
Toll Free 1 800 81 7340 (Malaysia)
orders.singapore@partridgepublishing.com

www.partridgepublishing.com/singapore

# Contents

# Dedication

This book is dedicated to my Mother.
Who has inspired, motivated and supported me
in every endeavor of my life.
She has been my muse,
mentor and best friend.
With love to Ammi.


This book is also dedicated to my lovely nieces and
nephews –the brightest young people anyone could imagine.
I hope this book will inspire them to learn, and to make
a difference – personally, locally and globally.

# Preface

*"For I dipped into the future, far as human eye could see.*
*Saw the vision of the world, and all the wonder that would be."*
*~ Alfred Tennyson*

The turn of this century has brought us to the edge of an amazing new discovery. The biggest revolution medical science has ever seen is upon us. No doubt the advent of the vaccination by Edward Jenner and the discovery of penicillin by Alexander Fleming, advanced new ways of thinking about diseases and new means to protect us from them, however, the discovery of healing cells throughout our bodies, even in areas previously believed to be incapable of regeneration, as well as our ability to stimulate, expand and harness their healing potential, is poised to change medicine as we know it. Not only will this change the face of medicine, it will also improve the health status of millions who would have otherwise suffered for years and lived a poor quality of life.

The impact on humanity is expected to be so enormous and the ramifications so massive, that at this point we are incapable of making even a fair estimate of its full sway. The next decade could provide proof that will ultimately change our view of health, disease and treatment. People, who are in the know and understand this potential, acknowledge that this will not merely be an enhancement of the current medical treatment protocols; this will be a drastic departure to a new paradigm of health assessment, health maintenance and methods of treatment.

However, instead of celebrating this gift of nature, battle lines have been drawn. Everyone wants their view point to be respected and accepted without giving the same respect to opposing views. Stem cells, a potential harbinger of health and healing have become four letter words which, depending on their use, can incite passionate, even violent responses. As if this wasn't enough, within the scientific community itself, mentioning the promise of stem cells to offer "cure" for untreatable diseases of today results in an incensed and indignant reaction. I realize that we are not able to guarantee anything but I also don't see any harm in aiming high, and staying optimistic. Anticipating a cure is not misleading, it is encouraging hope. As long as we are actively working towards "finding a cure" and not, "not finding a cure" the probability of finding one remains higher.

In this book I will take you on a journey inwards - to the small organelles of a living cell, then further inside the nucleus, the chromosome, the gene, the DNA, all the way to the nitrogen bases that form the DNA and then travel back with you outwards from a cell to the tissue that forms organs which organize into systems that compose the body. I will explain how we study genes, cells, drugs and their reactions in an organism; how we test and trial these cells and drugs in the lab and in clinics; how experimental treatment becomes evidence-based treatment; and who has control of this process?

Unlike most other discoveries or inventions, there is no specific date or event that heralded the dawn of this awareness and knowledge. It was rather a slow process, much like putting together a giant jigsaw puzzle, which holds the knowledge and information of immeasurable proportions. As with a puzzle that has thousands of small units, it takes ages to find and correctly place the first few pieces. But after painstakingly working through thousands of miniscule components you will get to a stage where it gets easier to locate and place the next piece and from where it keeps gaining momentum. Every next piece is faster to identify and easier to place, advancing the project towards completion. The process finally starts to make sense, at least in parts. The penultimate and ultimate pieces fall in place quickly and effortlessly, finally exposing the full picture with its articulate and prudent message of guidance. Once complete, it is bound to be a masterpiece for all to look at in awe, and drive the knowledge and benefits that it delivers.

Still, if one has to pin down some key pieces of this puzzle that allowed our progression to go faster and in the right direction, I would have to say they were:

1 - 1958: Dr. John Gordon cloned a tadpole with the genetic characteristics of the original frog.
2 - 1961: Dr. James Till and Ernest McCulloch proved stem cells exist.
3 - 1978: Dr Robert Edwards successfully delivered the first IVF baby, Louis J. Brown.
4 - 1981: Dr. Gail Martin isolated stem cells from mice embryo and Dr. Martin Evans grew them in a petri dish.
5 - 1996: Dr Ian Wilmut cloned the first mammal, Dolly the Sheep.
6 - 1998: Dr. James Thompson isolated the first human embryonic stem cells.
7 - 2006: Dr. Shinya Yamanaka reprogrammed adult cells into embryonic-like cells.
8 - 2008: Dr. Marius Werning and Dr. Deepak Srivastava directly reprogrammed adult mouse cells into heart and brain cells respectively. Dr. Mic Bhatia repeated the same feat with human cells.

In a span of only 50 years (1958 – 2008), we have gone from not even knowing the existence of stem cells embedded throughout our body, to being able to make practically any type of cell from a simple mature skin cell. Since then, work has progressed at a rapid pace and scientists have reprogrammed many adult cells directly into a variety of functional pluripotent cells. Now practically daily, samples of new disease cell lines, direct reprogramming of a variety of cells, new mechanisms of differentiation and development are being discovered and reported, filling in the gap of knowledge that existed even a decade ago.

Our bodies, since eternity, have housed magical cells previously believed to be the privilege of only fetuses. These amazing cells have been regenerating our bodies for millennia without any awareness or knowledge on our part. This book focuses on this gift we all have been bequeathed with at birth, and which stays with us from cradle to grave healing us from inside, day in and day out. However, until now we didn't know how to unlock this gift's potential to our best advantage. The perpetual increase in our knowledge in the stem cell field will ultimately open radical new doors leading to unmatched learning and unparalleled success in the treatment of previously untreatable conditions. Innovative means and approaches we haven't yet thought of, will likely become every day practice. Advancement and technology in this field is poised to catapult us into a sci-fi-like realm that may make today's medicine look primitive, within our life time. Within the foreseeable future we will very likely use one of the stem cell based therapies for a common or a serious illness. These will ultimately save many of us from the degenerative diseases that are a part and parcel of life.

As scientists in the last century started putting the pieces of this regenerative puzzle together, the progress initially was inevitably slow. Small, scattered bits of the picture that formed did not make much sense in isolation. However, as additional pieces became available (in vitro fertilization, animal cloning, embryonic cell lines, discovery of tissue stem cells, discovery of the plasticity of adult stem cells), the larger picture started to come in view and the excitement within the scientific community boosted the pace of discoveries. With every new discovery the recognition of this relationship between isolated pieces of information became more relatable. Every major breakthrough came with its own entourage of smaller relevant discoveries (converting blood cells into liver or pancreas cells, fat cells into cartilage or bone, etc.), filling in the gaps and imparting more colour and texture to the evolving picture. A new human organ system took shape and became recognized. I would call it "The MesoStromal Regeneration System". Mesoderm is the middle layer of the embryo from which blood, marrow and fat evolve and retain their stem cells. Stroma is the matrix that supports the cells and where the stem cells reside and on demand assist with tissue regeneration anywhere in the body. Together these components form the previously unrecognized healing system of the body. It slowly gained acceptance after numerous discoveries by a number of researchers were put together to complete the picture and profile of this complex system.

The central components of this system are the stem cells which possess the impressive properties of longevity, plasticity and self-replication. They can live for very long periods of time (longevity), can give rise to a variety of different cell types (plasticity), and can maintain their number by self-renewal. An average body cell does not enjoy any of these properties. The book you are holding is all about this potential that our stem cells retain and the important scientific and clinical questions that are being answered daily. We are getting closer to a day when we will learn the secret of regeneration and self-healing. This is our birthright and it's about time we claim its full benefits.

This book also has a larger mission; it aims to educate the masses about the real life benefits of stem cells, their nature, sources, and potential. It describes with clarity what everyone needs to know and understand before being influenced by any emotional or dogmatic argument against scientific progress. Clarifying the science and the facts behind the scene is at the core of this book. My goal is to help the reader pose the right questions and reach the correct answers. It is my sincere hope that it will encourage you to support the scientific advances in all possible directions, following appropriate ethical considerations, but not threatened by dogmatic or irrational beliefs.

New developments in the field of stem cell medicine have the potential to radically revise our understanding of health and healing. This book describes the natural state of stem cells, their role in health and disease and the ways this role can be supported, enhanced, expanded and scaled. It also describes clinical trials and stem cell uses in specific diseases as well as what the future holds for those who suffer from one of these awful ailments.

Current understanding of stem cell and tissue regeneration provides a pretty solid base of knowledge to build upon. When combined with the existing knowledge of the immune system and disease pathology, it tells us about healing under normal and diseased conditions. Studies in the lab, in animals and in humans, have provided scientists and doctors with deeper understanding of the differentiation potential, the reprogramming, and the non-cellular benefits of these cells.

With the passing of time, a detailed and more comprehensive picture is evolving filling the gaps between pieces with the glue of in-depth knowledge. New discoveries are detailing how during embryonic development, the turning on and off of genes in rapid succession, direct the primitive cells into one direction or the other. These cells then move to their pre-destined locations taking cues from surrounding cells and clues given by cell to cell contact and chemical signals. The same signals are now being used in the lab to reverse the march of any mature body cells back towards its embryonic identity, or to move one adult cell type into a distinctly different cell type.

*Why use bitter soup for healing, when sweet water is everywhere?*
*- Rumi*

Based on this knowledge, scientists and doctors are now testing these cells for the possible treatment of a variety of diseases. This approach has the potential to achieve a level of healing and cure for diseases that was never before considered possible. The challenge now is to perserve these promising opportunities, while continuing to question their veracity and long-term implications. It is also important to keep in mind that this particular field of research remains a delicate, balancing act between progresses, and skirting the legal and ethical traps scattered around the field. We must not let the fear of hurting few sensibilities get in the way of making millions of hopes and dreams become a reality.

No time has ever existed in isolation; the past is not detachable from the present and neither is the future. Today's research and its triumphs are rooted in the scientific advances of the 17th, 18th and 19th centuries and the medical progress of the 20th century. Unfortunately, the challenges and objections to this research are also rooted in our history, which may be a good place to learn. The science-religion debate and confrontation is age old. History has shown us occasion after occasion, no matter how intense the religious suppression, in the end the scientific truth was venerated and religions had to adopt accordingly. However, quite strangely we keep visiting the same arguments generation after generation, though in a different disguise.

We are on a journey; we haven't yet reached the destination. Many stops, many lessons, many discoveries, and many passions await us on this journey. What we learn and how we grow from these experiences will determine what the destination will mean to us. How we proceed with the medial advances and how we overcome the challenges, will dictate what the future of medicine will look like and how the quality and span of our lives will be impacted.

"Panacea in my veins" is intended for any reader who is interested in a better understanding of cellular biology, as it pertains to stem cells and healing. Anyone who wants to know what and where an answer for their ailment may lie might find guidance in the pages of this book. This book is for people who until now thought science and medicine is difficult to comprehend and make sense of. This is my endeavour to change that perception and 'cell by cell' breakdown the hard-to-understand concepts in a simple story-telling language.

I have attempted to correct some of the misconceptions and perhaps vent a little frustration with the way some special interest groups have retarded the progress of something that should have been a celebration for all of humanity. My work in the field of medicine in general, and rehabilitation and regeneration in particular, has provided me with some unforgettable conversations and unique experiences. It has taught me a great deal about human motivation, the source of their passion, and the deep impact that lack of knowledge has on people's perceptions and actions.

I have painstakingly added hundreds of references to all chapters of this book in the hope that it will lead the readers to explore further and find productive directions for the self-discovery of facts. It might also help readers identify reliable sources of scientific information from basic cell biology to cutting-edge clinical trials.

*Everything in the universe is within you. Ask all from yourself.*

*~ Rumi*

# Chapter 1

# INTRODUCTION

*"The important thing is not to stop questioning;*
*Curiosity has its own reason for existing."*
*~ Albert* Einstein.

The air felt sterile and warm, permeated with the smell of Silvadene cream, every now and then an alarm going off in the background. Staff hurriedly moved between beds and monitors, clad in disposable blue gowns, masks and caps, checking….adjusting…..dispensing…..comforting. The wails of the families from the hallway occasionally cut through the quiet of the ward. The typical smell of the burns, and the cries and moans of the victims are hard to erase from memory.

It was April 19, 1993. I was working as a resident physician in the burns ward of Parkland Memorial Hospital, Dallas. The 7 weeks siege at the Branch Davidian religious sect compound in Waco, Texas had just ended in a deadly fire. A number of survivors of the incident with both thermal and chemical burn injuries were brought in. Since then, everyday, burn dressing time was like re-living the acute burn injury as the wounds were unwrapped, cleaned and redressed. Despite every effort to minimize pain, control anxiety and to be gentle, the misery and the sense of helplessness remained palpable. Unfortunately that's just the nature of the injury and its consequences.

Few injuries are more horrific and few patients face more agonizing and longer recoveries than those with severe burns. It is one of the most painful injuries imaginable, mostly because when the skin burns it leaves the raw nerve endings exposed, causing severe pain. If a pin prick that is over less than a millimeter small can make you say"ouch!", then what must it be like to have 50% or 60% of one's body surface burned.

Even if one survives this stage of acute burns, the disfigurement, the non-healing wounds, and the multiple surgeries are such a nightmare that I wouldn't wish it even for my worst enemy. In today's medicine, the treatment of burns, after the life-saving efforts, is focused on the treatment of the wounds. Deep burns don't heal on their own, slices of skin from the remaining healthy skin have to be removed, then shredded to expand, stretched, and then surgically transplanted over the wound. The healing is slow and leaves mesh-like scars, contractures, chronic pain, disfiguring, pigmentation, and functional deformities. If all this sounds dreadful, that's because it is.

Now imagine a patient with burns comes in the emergency department. The doctor first numbs a small area of healthy skin, then takes a postage stamp-sized thin slice of skin, puts it in a chemical that turns it into liquid, which is then placed in a spray gun. In the meantime, the wounds are cleaned; the patient is hydrated and given pain medicines. This gun is ready to spray the patient's own stem cells from his/her skin on to the burns, covering an area about the size of a printer paper and heals in 5-7 days without any scar, pigmentation, or deformity. The patient walks out of the hospital a week later.

Sounds sci-fi? May be not.

Fifteen years after the Waco Branch Davidian compound fire, I was working in Australia when I first came in contact with this skin gun developed by scientist Marie Stoner and plastic surgeon Dr. Fiona Wood of Perth, Australia. (1) The skin spray gun has been in use in Australia since 1993. The technology is currently approved for use in Australia, Europe, Mexico, Canada and China but not yet in The United States of America, though it is now undergoing trials here as well. If you or a loved one needed this treatment and were told you cannot yet get it in the USA, though it has been in use in other developed countries for over a decade, would it make you furious? If it did, you won't be alone.

The "spray on skin" gun is just one example of the novel treatments that are being developed, based on stem cell science, and you don't have to kill any embryos, perform any abortions, buy a fetus on the black market or create hybrid monsters (as some of the stem cell opponents will have you believe), to obtain them. In fact you have stem cells hiding in every organ of your body. (2) They are working day and night to repair the billions of cells that are damaged in our bodies during the course of an honest day's work. If you want to know what is available and what is coming next in the stem cell arena, which would change the face of medicine, you need to stay abreast with the knowledge in this field and learn for yourself what is good for you and your loved ones. Be mindful to act when you need to, so that we don't let some corrupt pharmaceutical lobbyist, dishonest politician or religious fundamentalist take away this opportunity to alleviate human suffering, or make it so expensive that most of us will not be able to afford it.

In today's world, for many of us, just about everything is getting more convenient and accessible due to the advances in technology across almost all sectors. But have you ever considered why so many still fail to avail the full benefits of these advances? When other variables are accounted for, it is not the lack of resources, or the limit to access, or even the inability to use them, but mostly the lack of knowledge of their existence and the lack of information about where to access them.

As a physician, I have often been surprised as to how many people do not know the benefits, options, services and provisions they have accessible to them, in their healthcare plan, at their healthcare provider or with their employer. When asked why they are not taking advantage of those benefits, the universal answer is, "I didn't know about them".

For many of us there exists a gap between what we know and what it will take to reap the benefits of the knowledge and technology that is available to us. This book is an effort to bridge that gap. I therefore propose that for the sake of better health and better healthcare, learning about our bodies and our healthcare system is everyone's responsibility. When it comes to challenging topics like stem cells, their life and health-saving benefits, funding for their research and the politics involved, it is crucial that we all are well-informed. We need to see, feel, learn for ourselves, and refuse to be misled by special interest groups, ignorant politicians and close-minded professionals.

*"Few is the number of those who think with their own mind
and feel with their own heart".*
*- Albert Einstein*

The science of medicine is sometimes made out to be too difficult to understand or too complex to comprehend. In today's reality it is neither that complex nor that out of reach. All you need is a simply laid out, honest and accurate explanation by the writer, and an open mind by the reader and we can all be on the same page.

Any idea or discovery, no matter how groundbreaking, needs to reach a certain level of consciousness to make its mark. In order to bring about a paradigm shift in old thinking and practice, this information must be disseminated to a critical tipping position where it can raise the level of awareness to the point of bearing fruit. This is imperative, to avoid the risk of being ignored or suppressed.

Suppressed? You ask. Yes! Every new idea, innovation, invention and discovery has its skeptics, opponents, enemies and agents whose job it is to resist change. Human history is replete with such examples. Unfortunately, we only hear about the successes that made it despite these oppositions; past the claims of heresay, that rose above the mockery of their peers, and survived the fires at the stake and beheadings at the guillotine. I often wonder how much of human advancement we left buried at those sites, perished under the oppression of the draconian laws of the day.

Understanding the mystery of life is one of the most exciting and remarkable areas of science to explore. Knowledge about biology, disease and medicine allows a better knowhow of our bodies, in health and in disease. It is, therefore, in the interest of everyone to better understand our cellular and genetic makeup and how disease and injury affect it.

Most of us take our health for granted, but ask anyone who suffers from an untreatable, chronic or disabling illness, and you would realize how precious health really is. The reality is that every one of us will face some kind of illness; everyone will grow old and die. Fortunate are those who will have access to better healthcare and better treatment options than we do today. Cellular and regenerative medicine, based on stem cells, holds such a promise.

In today's medicine, very often, we have the diagnostic tools to find what is wrong or damaged in a particular disease. Our treatment options though, are limited to the relief of symptoms in most cases, with the exception of infectious diseases for which we have antibiotics. Even this is not true in the case of viral infections or drug-resistant bacteria. After decades of medical learning, research, and technological advancement, we are nowhere near a cure to most ailments.

> *"The life so short, the craft so long to learn."- Hippocrates.*

However, it is impressive when you realize that as many, or even more diseases, are self-limiting and resolved by the body's own disease-fighting apparatus without any treatment. It reminds me of Voltaire.

> *"The art of medicine consists in amusing the patient*
> *while nature cures the disease."- Voltaire*

Health, therefore, is a delicate play between the rate at which a disease, causes damage to our cells and the body's ability to heal and restore itself. This fight between our adversaries and our bodies is an ongoing battle in which our health hangs in the balance. Nature, through evolution, has equipped our bodies with tools and ways to fight a myriad of diseases and foreign organisms that mean us harm. The system however, is not foolproof for it sometimes misses the target, is misled into attacking the wrong target or is simply not strong enough to handle the threat.

**Science and Nature:**

As old as human history may be, nature never ceases to amaze us by giving up some of its secrets every now and then. In fact, scientific discoveries are nothing but the observation of nature. All major discoveries in science came from a deeper observation of nature. (3) No one invented gravity, or buoyancy or anomalous expansion of water. We learned all these by observation. Whether it was major advancements such as the flight of a plane or something as simple as

Velcro, they are all derivatives of a deeper observation of nature. *Edward Jenner* observed immunity to small pox by exposure to cow pox, while *Alexander Fleming* observed the inability of bacteria to grow on a dish contaminated by penicillin producing fungus. (4)

> *The art of healing comes from nature, not from the physician.*
> *Therefore the physician must start from nature, with an open mind.*
> *~ PhilipusAureolus Paracelsus*

Similar medical observations in the last decade gave us an understanding and a clue to a natural healing system that has the potential to alleviate the sufferings of millions of humans. This discovery is the existence of functional stem cells in living humans with their ability to repair damaged cells by stimulating or becoming almost any type of cell. They can reach and help repair dead or damaged tissues in practically every organ system of the human body. (5)

We have had many lifetimes to get used to nature, technology on the other hand is fairly new. Often people, who understand technology or science well, are not always as proficient in explaining it to others. Technology can be daunting, and even frustrating, to understand, mostly because it is not explained or described well for easy comprehension. With the escalating difficulty of understanding, we build a wall, reinforced by our feelings of inadequacy. This in turn, can spark a feeling of unease and mistrust. When we give something a fair go but cannot figure it out, it is natural to get cognitively discouraged, to shy away and eventually be content to follow and trust the alleged and vocal experts in the field.

I intend to change that; here I will, cell by cell, breakdown the complex structures, processes and experiments related to stem cells, so it is simple, easy and interesting for all to understand. Readers may make their own decision about how things ought to progress and what should or should not be supported by publicly-funded research. I only want to encourage every person to take an active role in the future care and management of their own bodies.

> *"All censorships exist to prevent anyone from challenging current conceptions*
> *and existing institutions. All progress is initiated by challenging current*
> *conceptions, and executed by supplanting existing institutions."*
> *~ George Bernard Shaw.*

## Science and Faith:

Although times have changed, human emotions and deep-rooted beliefs—whether philosophical, political, or spiritual—that underlie the opposition of medical advancement and technology have remained relatively consistent. The fact also remains that attitudes, beliefs, and religious establishments do eventually come around when scientific facts can no longer be refuted. Public opinion does eventually sway in favor of new technology when personal need or tragedy hits closer to home and results in a newer more personal perspective of the point in question.

What is it that brings about that tipping point? I believe it is the critical mass of credible, well-informed and literate people in society that elevate the overall consciousness about a particular technology, development or discovery. Then and only then, it reaches the stage where it is accepted, adopted and appreciated.

> *"Truth, in its struggle for recognition, passes through four distinct stages.*
> *First, we say it is damnable, dangerous, disorderly, and will surely*
> *disrupt society. Second, we declare it is heretical, infidelic and contrary*
> *to the Bible. Third, we say it is a matter of no importance one way or the*
> *other. Fourth, we aver that we have always upheld and believed it".*
> *American philosopher, Elbert Hubbard.*

My goal with this book is to educate the general public of the facts, and warn them of the fiction purported as fact, relating to the nature and potential of stem cells—not only embryonic but also their own adult stem cells—to understand the benefit that can be achieved by exploring and studying them fully, without limitations and restrictions, and protecting them from special interest groups, as well as religious and political rhetoric.

It is important to achieve this goal, because this is, without a doubt, the most significant and revolutionary discovery for treating illness and disease. A true scientific revolution—this being the dawn of a new, modern approach to health and healing—which is destined to change the way medicine has been practiced over the centuries. (6) If left to the devices of the political and pharmaceutical profit mongers, humanity may miss out on the biggest medical breakthrough of the century if not the millennium.

Current information on stem cell and regenerative medicine is often too piecemeal and unengaging, or just grossly exaggerated, often poorly laid out, and even more often shrouded in political, religious and commercial agendas making it hard to navigate through. The confusing jargon or sometimes intentional, misleading statements make it hard to find unbiased third-party sources of information. On top of that, we have a healthcare system that is not primed to incorporate these advances, either from a technical and logistical standpoint or from an intellectual one. It is becoming increasingly clear that this field will have many more challenges without knowledgeable healthcare providers, patients, and other stakeholders. I hope this message will reach many who ought to learn and get involved in the fight for the cure of diseases that cause immeasurable human suffering.

I also want to extend hope, through this book, to those who are, or whose loved ones are suffering from serious or disabling illnesses for which there is little hope today. Strength of humanity is not in giving up. Often there is a way, if we can look hard and look in the right place. So look keenly here and you may find directions to the right place; to a valley of hope where you may discover the miracle by finally realizing and learning that you, yourself are the miracle.

*In vain have you acquired knowledge,*
*if you do not impart knowledge onto others.*

# Chapter 2

# HISTORY OF DISEASE

*"The aim of medicine is to prevent disease and prolong life, the ideal of medicine is to eliminate the need of a physician."~ William James mayo*

Modern medicine has its origins deep in the ancient world. Sickness and disease has been a part of human existence since time immemorial. The history of sickness and its treatment started out with beliefs in supernatural causes and the use of herbs and potions for treating the sick and afflicted. Religion and magic frequently played a role in attempted healing and perceived protection from disease.

In ancient Greece, besides general gods of healing like Apollo, there were also dedicated gods of health - Asklepios, Panakeia and Hygieia. Of these, the last one can be traced as far back as the 7th century BC, and even today we have inherited her name in words like hygiene. Greeks were not alone in keeping health gods. Egyptian goddess Isis Medica, and the Roman Bona Dea had similar occupations. (1,2)

With intellectual evolution, experience and observation, we gradually overcame some of these superstitions. Better and more authentic means of diagnosis and treatment, based on scientific facts, became popular. The important point to note, however, is that at any given time the accepted means of medical practice or the stated "standards of care" were furiously defended by its practitioners, no matter how blatantly wrong they were by today's standards.

It is a shame to see that the close-minded and arrogant approach of some healthcare practitioners or health administrators has not changed over the centuries. In fact, in some ways, it has become worse, partly confounded by secondary gain, conflict of interest and trillions of dollars in the mix. The resultant intensity of arguments beats any historical controversy.

Relating health to God's grace and sickness to personal morality is not a new thought. In the Judeo-Christian tradition, sickness has often been seen as a divine punishment for sin. History is rife with examples of the self-righteous people criticizing treatment of many diseases—especially sexually transmitted diseases like syphilis—associating them with encouragement of immoral behavior. Not much has changed in some circles, even today.

> *"AIDS is not just God's punishment for homosexuals; it is God's punishment for the society that tolerates homosexuals." -Jerry Falwell.*

Neither the focus of this book nor its capacity will allow me to discuss the ludicrousness and absurdity of this thought process, but the fact remains that it is as old as medicine itself. Before we start exposing the absurd arguments and devious ways special interest groups mislead the public about stem cell research and its potential, let us briefly take a trip to the beginning of organized medicine and its theories that reined the thought and practice of medicine for centuries, only to be proven wrong in its entirety.

Hippocrates (ca. 460–370 BC) has been associated with the first central principle of western medicine the "Humoral theory of disease" that influenced medical practices from antiquity through the 19th century.(3)

> *Your theory is crazy, but it's not crazy enough to be true.*
> *~Niels Bohr*

According to this defunct theory the "humor" or "fluid" in the human body is divided into four distinct types. Black bile, yellow bile, blood, and phlegm. Each individual was believed to have a certain humoral makeup, and health was defined as the proper humoral balance; an imbalance was considered the cause of all diseases. The same four humors also referred to the four different individual psychological temperaments: melancholic, choleric, sanguine, and phlegmatic. Each of these humors was associated with the seasons, and each was considered as having the qualities of hotness, coldness, wetness and dryness. It was believed that since an individual's humoral balance was connected with other phenomena—such as sex, age, social class, diet, climate, geographic location, occupation and even planetary alignment—the same could not apply to all and what was good for one might not be so for another. Recommended treatments included bloodletting, vomits, enemas, purges and abstinence from sex.

Bloodletting was closely associated with the humoral theory as a common treatment modality and was practiced with varying intensity by different practitioners (4) for the treatment of a number of diseases. The two key concepts pertaining to bloodletting were the false belief that blood was created and then used up—it did not circulate; so it could stagnate—and that it was related to the humoral balance, both of these concepts we now know to be incorrect.

After Hippocrates, this theory was elaborated further by Galen in the second century and developed even further by Arabic and European scholars for centuries to follow, not however, due to lack of challenges. Andreas Vesalius's *De Humani Corporis Fabrica* in 1543 and William Harvey's *De Motu Cordis* in 1628 challenged parts of the humoral theory. The establishment, however, maintained it to be the dominant concept among both physicians and the public through the 19th century.(5)

Today even a preschooler can tell you that bugs can make you sick and not even a lay person on the street will buy into Hippocrates humoral theory of disease much less a healthcare practitioner. Do realize that for centuries the practitioners of the day not only practiced but defended it and ridiculed anyone who challenged the status quo, much less offer an idea like the germ theory of disease.

The history of the world is full of similar stories of scholars and doctors defending their practices and blindly following the established experts in the field no matter how deeply wrong they were. Nicholas Copernicus, around 1515, composed a manuscript, entitled "Commentariolus", suggesting that the sun was the center of the planetary motions, thus challenging the millennia old geocentric belief of the time.(6) Contemporaries of Copernicus, including liberals like Martin Luther, denounced the Copernican system in favor of the commonly accepted geocentric view of his day. Others like Tycho Brahe presented his own schemes, observationally equivalent to that of Copernicus. In his rendition, the moon and sun revolved around a stable earth while the other planets circled the sun, thus conveniently staying in the good graces of the church and partially staying true to science.

Even in 1616, when Galileo Galilei became a defender of the Copernican system, he was summoned to Rome, tried by the Inquisition and found guilty of heresay. Galileo was then forced to recant his Copernican belief thus making sure the established geocentric concept persisted. If you think this happened only in the ancient times and it's easier to challenge the established schools of thought and belief now, think again.

The eighteenth century has been called the age of enlightenment or the age of reason, but even during the 18th century attitudes did not change much at all. You may recall that, in 1747, Dr. James Lind, an officer and naval surgeon in the British Royal Navy, established the fact that oranges and lemons were effective in curing scurvy.(7) Lind divided patients into 6 groups and gave each group a different remedy. Only the group given oranges and lemons recovered. (8) Based on his observations he recommended the use of lemons to prevent the disease in the sailors. It took Lind 41 years to convince the British Royal Navy to implement his recommendation; thereafter, the incidence of scurvy among the British sailors sharply declined.

Today we know that the smallpox vaccination has helped eradicate this horribly lethal and disfiguring disease. But in the early 1800's when Edward Jenner's cowpox experiments showed that he could protect a child from smallpox if he infected the kid with lymph from a cowpox blister, his ideas were met with immediate criticism by other healthcare practitioners, clergy and the public in general.(9) The rationale for this criticism varied, from sanitary, religious, scientific, to political objections.

Demonstrators in UK, led elaborate anti-vaccination marches, complete with banners, a child's coffin, and an effigy of Jenner.(10) The Catholic Church was just as opposed until the next wave of smallpox killed droves of Catholics while many Protestants who vaccinated survived. This gradually changed the church's hard stance. Towards the end of the 19<sup>th</sup> century, smallpox outbreaks in the United States led to anti-vaccine campaigns here at home with equally strong rhetoric—despite the already established proof of benefits documented by the practice in Britain. Unfortunately even today in some parts of the world, people resist vaccination and react violently against the international healthcare workers providing such life-saving vaccinations.

Examining the history of a more recent medical practice, blood transfusion runs a fair parallel to stem cell challenges. This life-saving treatment ran a similar course that the medical use of stem cell is facing today. The history of blood transfusion is ironically quite bloody. 17<sup>th</sup> century Europe was abuzz with excitement over the possibility of blood transfusion. Both English and French scientists were in a race to get there first, and animal experiments and theoretical debates preceded animal to human transfusions with mostly disastrous results. Instead of allowing regulated and controlled scientific experimentation, the resistance and objections to transfusions, mostly religious, resulted in the practice being banned for over a century.

Many 17<sup>th</sup> century politicians and physicians believed that science was toying with forces of nature and working against the perceived will of God. It is this same argument that has come back to hinder progress century after century. Power brokers, who were against transfusions, raised fears that transfusions will transmute animal qualities or personal characteristics from the donor to the recipients resulting in monstrous hybrid creatures. They went as far as claiming it will irreversibly corrupt the human race. Had it not been for this opposition to human blood transfusion, refinement of the technique and research would have had earlier success and likely prevented the loss of countless lives over that century.

This 17<sup>th</sup> century obsession was no less alive in 20<sup>th</sup> century America, where racial segregation made its way to the blood banks. In 1941, American Red Cross refused to accept African-American blood donations. In 1942, under criticism, the Red Cross did start accepting these donors but made it clear that the "colored" blood will be stored separately.(13)

All this was done in the absence of any clear scientific evidence. The events and stories of that era clearly proved that it was ignorance, not science, which was the reason behind such decisions. Proponents of segregation voiced concerns such as the fear of having a black child after a "colored" blood transfusion, destruction of the purity of blood lines, or birth of a deformed offspring.

It was not that long ago...we are talking of 1959 USA. Two decades passed in this ignorance, but instead of getting better, the debate reached a new worse when Dr. John Scudder and his friends used unscientific and deceptive case reports, presented as proof of race mismatched blood transfusion, to be the cause of serious complications. This was nothing more than ignorance and racism on the part of these physicians. With their pseudo-scientific data in hand and their racist comrades by their side, they argued for a race-based blood donor selection protocol. Scudder's claims got a lot of publicity despite the fact that other physicians in the country working in academic institutions made their disagreement to Scudder publicly known. More interestingly, there was clearly no basis for these claims since the South African Red Cross had confirmed interracial blood transfusions to be safe. This was on the basis of data on interracial transfusions performed in their country for more than 20 years without any known adverse effects.

Many scientific studies and reports since then confirmed that there was no advantage or scientific basis for intra-racial over inter-racial transfusion. But would it surprise you that despite the objective evidence from local as well as the international scientific community, practice of blood segregation based on race in some of the southern states continued well into the 1970s?

Imagine someone with pneumonia being treated with a lit candle inside a glass, placed on the patient's back. This was the accepted treatment for pneumonia before the advent of penicillin. I don't have to tell you how ridiculous it sounds today. Suffering caused by organ failure, post-transplant complications, and the use of toxic medications, may appear equally primitive in the near future if the stem cell treatments reach the potential that many scientists believe they hold.

My reason to go over this remote and not so remote history of medicine is to make the reader aware how distortion of the facts in order to support certain political or religious beliefs has been a constant in human history. If you observe with an open mind you will see the same prejudices at work today.

What is at stake today is larger than one race or one country. The problem is that science gathers knowledge faster than society gathers wisdom.

The United States has been the leader in biomedical technology and medical research for more than a century. The lack of adequate funding for proper research, ideological barriers to advancement of science and criminalization of scientific innovation is stifling scientific thought. Not only has this led to the loss of leadership in this field to other nations, but the dearth of scientific research and advancement in the USA has held back the world scientific community in advancing stem cell science. Not to mention the many small nations which do not have the resources to set their own scientific and ethical policies or strategies follow our lead. It is therefore imperative that we learn, understand and act in time, to claim our right to the best cures nature has to offer, and also help advance the biggest revolution in the history of medicine. I don't want any of us to be left behind, to suffer unnecessarily, or die without taking advantage of one of the best solutions for human healing and restoration.

I invite you to read the following chapters with an open mind, feel free to evaluate the facts and look up the references to learn and know for yourself what is fact, and what is fiction. See through the sensationalized statements with no medical basis, claims that "there is proof" when no such established scientific proof exists.

You have a choice; believe in the established wisdom, dogma and views of a small vocal minority and their deeply entrenched personal beliefs, or enhance your own knowledge. You are free to refuse that the earth is round, the planets revolve around the sun, or that there are other universes. You can deny that vaccination can protect against infectious diseases or that you can safely accept a matched blood transfusion from another race. But if you want to use your own intelligence and trust the process of scientific peer-reviewed research and can keep an open mind, then tighten your seatbelt and read on. The ride into the world of human biology, its intricate process of self-preservation and the potential to use this knowledge for the benefit of the human race is wildly exhilarating.

# Chapter 3

# THE CELL

*"Man is a microcosm, or a little world, because he is an extract from all the stars and planets of the whole firmament, from the earth and the elements; and so he is their quintessence" ~ Philipus Aureolus Paracelsus*

If man is a microcosm, the cell is an even smaller version of this microcosm. There are several theories about the origin of life on primitive earth. It may have arrived on earth via meteorites, created in deep-sea vents, or synthesized by lightning in a reducing atmosphere. There is no objective proof which defines what the first self-replicating life form was. Cells emerged at least 3.5 billion years ago. (1) These were simple in constitution and evolved over time into more complex structures.

Regardless of what the origin of life may have been, nature starts all life with the development of a single cell. This cell may evolve into more and more complex organisms or stay content as a unicellular organism. Though it may increase in complexity, the basic components remain the same. It is therefore crucial to understand the microcosm of a cell which represents the basic structure and function of all living creatures.

Just as the invention of the telescope made the cosmos more accessible to observation, the microscope opened up new vision of the smaller worlds. In 1665, Robert Hooke noticed small spaces in cork under his microscope which represented dead cell walls but looked like small quarters where the monks used to live, spaces called "cellula". These microscopic spaces were thus named

"Cells". Later Anton Van Leeuwenohek, in 1674, examined and described the detailed contents of a cell, using his own rendition of the microscope.

Evolution of science and the study of living organisms over the years has established the cell as the basic unit of structure and function in all living things, sometimes called the 'building blocks' of life. All living cells are surrounded by a cell membrane and contain a nucleus, in which genetic material or chromosomes are housed. In between the nucleus and the cell membrane is the cytoplasm, which is fluid in nature, and contains many small structures or organelles, some of which have their own membranes and many of these are believed to have different evolutionary origins. These organelles perform a variety of functions necessary for the survival of the cell.

Earliest life started as single cells and many of these bacteria, amoebae and algae still exist and share the same basic structure with other living cells. More complex organisms are made of progressively increasing number of cells leading up to human beings where they number around 37 trillion cells. What is interesting is that another 100 trillion microbes, mostly single-cell organisms, reside in and on a human body. This approximately 1000 species strong collection of microrganisms is called a "microbiome" which plays a very important role in keeping an individual healthy and functioning well.

In complex organisms like humans there are more than 200 different types of cells. These cells have a number of structural and functional differences but similar basic properties. A cell, though small, is a complex structure, its cytoplasm studded with multiple small organelles, resemble in function to the human organs at a miniature scale... the cell membrane for transport, protection and covering, cytoskeleton to help maintain cell shape and movement, lysosomes to digest, ribosomes to perform protein and lipid syntheses, Golgi apparatus for packaging and releasing concentrated proteins and lipids; vacuoles to transport the finished proteins and lipids; microtubules for internal support; centrioles to operate the cellular division and cellular reproduction, while mitochondria to produce and supply energy for all of these activities.

Mitochondria are unique in the sense that besides the nucleus they are the only other site in the cell that contains genetic material or DNA. An interesting fact about this additional DNA is that unlike chromosomal DNA which comes half from a mother and half from a father, all of the mitochondrial DNA always comes from the mother (remember this important fact for later discussions or to send your kids on a guilt trip). The mitochondria are believed to have been small primitive bacteria that invaded the budding cell life at some stage of evolution. They survived endocytosis (being ingested by the cell). Later these ingested bacteria got incorporated in the cell itself and built a symbiotic relationship that has lasted for millennia. Unlike other organelle, mitochondria originate only from other mitochondria. They contain their own circular DNA, along with their own transcription tools, much like other bacteria in nature. (2)

The most prominent structure in a cell is the nucleus or the brain of the cell. In humans the nucleus contains 46 chromosomes, (44 somatic and 2 sex chromosomes--either X or Y) each of which is made of one long strand of DNA. 23 of these chromosomes come from the father and 23 from the mother. Together these chromosomes make pairs and represent our genetic blueprint. The total amount of DNA in each cell contains all the information needed to create a complete individual. Though the same amount of DNA is present in each cell, the entire code is not functioning in every cell and only a selected part of the DNA information is active in different types of cells, thus maintaining the differentiations in each category of cells. For example, a liver cell is different from a muscle cell which is different from a skin cell in size, shape and function but carries the exact same content of DNA.

The DNA is composed of a sugar backbone, "Deoxyribose" which is studded with nitrogen bases creating the "Deoxyribonucleic Acid" (DNA). The four nitrogen bases found in DNA are A (adenine), C (cytosine), G (guanine), T (thymine). Together these nitrogen bases or nucleotides form a complementarity pairing system where guanine and cytosine exclusively bond with each other (G:C), and so do adenine and thymine (A:T). Together this monogamous interaction of nucleotides strengthened by hydrogen bonds creates the stable double-strand of DNA. A series of these bases, each of variable length, constitutes a gene; we have about 23,000 of these gene sequences in our DNA. (3)

Each amino acid in a protein is represented by a codon of 3 consecutive nucleotides. Each gene puts together a string of codons for a specific protein molecule. A long string of these codons, in a series, creates one of the strands of DNA while a second strand twists around the first with the help of its complementary paired bases. The structure of DNA thus consists of two strands of nucleotides that form a spiral ladder-like structure. One strand of DNA is the template from which the other one is built.

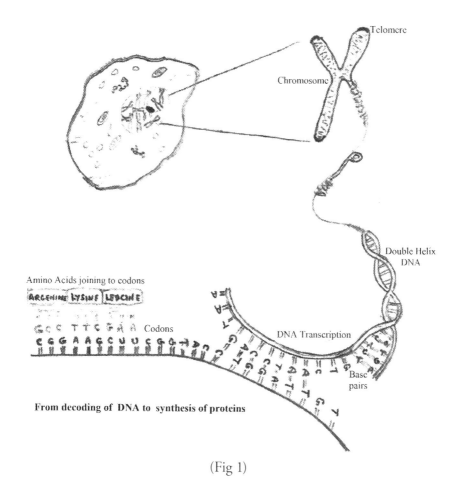

(Fig 1)

This double strand model was first described by Watson and Crick's Nobel Prize winning "Double Helix" DNA. This entire Double Helix structure, in turn, wraps around a special type of protein called histone. Histones serve to protect and prevent the entanglement of the long strands of DNA and allows for easier unzipping and zipping of the required area of a strand to make copies as needed. (4)

Through a series of steps (greatly simplified in the description below), when a particular protein is needed to be manufactured, the section of DNA where that particular protein gene resides, unzips; complementary bases attach to the open strand creating an RNA strand, which runs down the base sequences until it reaches a stop sign on the gene at which point it detaches as a single strand of RNA, the DNA then zips back up.

The messenger RNA (mRNA) now carries a series of codons, (3 bases each). Maintaining this sequence, it delivers this template to the ribosome where one of the 20 amino acids, corresponding to each codon on the template, is attached like a string of pearls. This synthesizes a protein molecule, ready to perform the function it is destined for.

If we assume that mRNA is composed of the following codons then this mRNA will code for a unique protein molecule. The genes, the mRNA and their resulting proteins can range in length from a few hundred to a few thousand nucleotides. (Each 3 base codon signifies 1 amino acid)

| ACC | GAU | CUA | GAU | AAA | CUA | GAGAGAGAG |
|------|---------|--------|---------|--------|--------|--------------|
| Arginine | Alanine | Lucien | Alanine | Valine | Lucien | End sequence |

(*These codes &sequences are for explanation only and not for exact representation*)

There are mechanisms in place to control which genes are to be activated for RNA production, which ones are to remain silent or permanently asleep, what amount of mRNA is to be produced and at what rate. The mRNA eventually undergoes degradation in order to prevent overproduction of any given protein. These mechanisms called epigenetic regulation are complex and responsible for controlling all genes in a particular stage of embryonic or fetal development keeping them either active or no longer accessible for transcription.

Defects or abnormalities at any stage in this complex process can have serious consequences. Simple substitution, deletion or addition of even a solitary base can result in a widely misread message. Very slight changes can result in major change in meanings (therapist vs the rapist; notable vs not able)...you get the jest.

Imagine deleting the first Adenine base (A) from the top row sequence in the example below. (See the result on lower part of the table)

| ACC | GAU | CUA | GAU | AAA | CUA | GAGAGAGA |
|------|------|------|------|------|------|------|
| Arginine | Alanine | Leucine | Alanine | Valine | Lucien | End sequence |
| A̶CCG | AUC | UAG | AUA | AAC | UAG | AGAGAGA |
| Glycine | Proline | Serine | Phenyl | tyrosine | Methionin | End sequence |

(*These codes &sequences are for explanation only and not for exact representation*)

Missing the first "A" from the original top sequence, changed all the codons on the bottom template and therefore the protein manufactured from this template will have a drastically different sequence of amino acids and hence a completely different protein molecule.

For example, in sickle cell anemia the genetic mutation is a single change in the amino acid building blocks of the oxygen-transport protein, hemoglobin. The beta-globin chain of the hemoglobin, in sickle cell disease has the amino acid valine at position 6 instead of the normal glutamic acid, this result in an abnormal hemoglobin molecule which disrupts the normal development of red blood cells and increases their destruction. A shortage of red blood cells or anemia prevents delivery of oxygen to the body's tissues thus leads to poor growth, organ damage, and other health problems. This shows how the substitution of even one amino acid can have devastating clinical consequences on the health of a patient.

When normal cells divide in the body or are grown in a petri dish they can only divide for a limited number of times even under optimal growth conditions. This limit on how many times cells can divide is called the Hayflick limit. When cells are grown in a culture, the young cells initially reproduce and divide rapidly making copies. As the cells age, this rate of division slows down and eventually stops. Once the cells lose the ability to divide or reach senescence, they undergo a programmed cellular death called apoptosis. The reason for this limit is that the well-defined ends of the DNA (telomeres) that prevent its fraying are shortened with each division of the cell. The telomeres are eventually, completely used up, at which point each cell reaches a stage of senescence and can no longer divide into daughter cells. (5)

There are two major exceptions to this scenario where the telomeres are able to maintain their length and function by restoring themselves with the help of an enzyme called telomerase. Telomerase is only found in stem cells and cancer cells, thus giving both of these cell types the ability to divide for an unlimited number of times without suffering from senescence.

Telomere can thus be considered a biological clock. (6) Their damage or shortening may be the reason for aging which is proportionate to the rate of loss of telomere length. There are families that have genetically long telomeres and associated history of longevity as well as medical conditions with short telomeres leading to pronounced rapid aging. One such disease is progeria, in which the child is born with defective or short telomeres causing rapid aging and death.

Human or animal cells can be grown artificially outside the body, mostly for the purpose of experimentation. Despite the fact that current cell culture methods permit maintenance of only limited cell types, biotechnological advances continue to provide opportunities and new cell lines are constantly being introduced. (7)

## POWER OF A CELL

*"You are not a drop in the ocean.*
*You are the entire ocean in a drop." — Rumi*

Every journey starts with the first step and that step in the journey of life is a cell. According to the evolution of life it all started with the first cell, a single cell which is like an ocean concealed in a drop. Hard to see even under a microscope, it has all the potential to make a 6 ft. tall human or a 600 lbs. gorilla. If that's just one cell, then imagine what trillions of cells in hundreds of varieties that make our body can potentially do, if we only knew how to unlock their full potential.

The idea of curing illness or injury by transplanting tissues, or organs, is as old as the history of medicine. Accounts of attempted bone transplant date back for centuries; Gaspare Tagliacozzi in the 16th century has been credited with skin transplant to fix disfiguring battle wounds. Even in ancient times, physicians knew that tissues from another person are rejected by the recipient of the graft. They learned from experience that for a skin graft to work it needed to come from the same person or be "autologous", and not from some other person or be "allogeneic".

As the knowledge of the immune system and tissue science advanced, we learned more about the way our body recognizes its own and rejects foreign tissues. Initial transplant experiences were in animals. Later successful human transplantation of bone, skin and corneas made advances in the 1920s. However, it wasn't until 1954, that Dr. Joseph Murray performed the first successful kidney transplant; its success was based on the fact that the donor and recipient were identical twins. In 1967, a South African heart surgeon, Christian Bernard, performed the first human heart transplant in Cape Town.

Further studies paved the way to test for matching tissues, control of rejection and survival of transplanted organs. The major problem remained to be the tendency of the body's immune system to reject the "foreign" organ. In order to prevent rejection, patients were given immune-suppressing medications. The first effective immunosuppressive drug Cyclosporine was introduced in 1978 which allowed better control of rejection. Other similar and less toxic drugs have since been developed. (More on this is in the transplant chapter)

While difficulties remained in using another person's tissues, transplant of autologous (patient's own) tissue continued to advance. In the first chapter we talked about skin transplant for burn patients where a surgeon borrows skin from one part of the body to cover the burned skin in another area. Similarly taking a small piece of a tendon to repair a ligament in the knee joint has also been routinely practiced for years. Another common surgical application is the use of a piece of the hip bone as a fill-in for spine surgery. Many of these tissues can also be taken from a cadaver or tissue bank with some caveats.

Despite success in autologous procedures, the problem of allogeneic transplant is still not solved and therefore it is important to understand this concept of the body's self-recognition and defense system. It is crucial to know and understand how and why stem cells or any other cells for that matter cannot just be transferred from one person to another willy-nilly. This will also explain the risks one takes if such a transfer is carried out without proper medical care and consideration.

As an individual organism, unique in countless ways, each human is made up of some 37 trillion cells put together in a very well organized fashion making tissues, organs and functional systems like the cardiovascular, digestive, respiratory, genitourinary, nervous, locomotive, hormonal, and last but not the least, the immune system. The body needs protection from chemical threats like acid or poison, environmental threats like fire or water, mechanical dangers like a knife or a nail and biological threats from organisms like bacteria, viruses, fungi, parasites, allergens and even insect or animal bites.

If the body is attacked in any manner, all different systems play a role in the protection and escape from that threat. However, once an agent penetrates and invades the body, the immune system bears the main responsibility to protect us. From the time of the first attack, depending on the route of invasion, the immune cells in the skin, lung or intestine, tackle the foreign invader and try to wrestle and subdue it. White blood cells play a major role in this battle, and a variety of these cells each have a unique function.

How do the white blood cells (WBC) know which cell is foreign? That's a very interesting question. Just like our facial features, finger prints, and retina images, our cells also have unique identification markers and no two humans (except identical twins) have the exact same markers. A body, therefore, can differentiate a friend from a foe on the basis of what identification it carries. Each cell has a number of markers on its surface that not only indicate the cell lineage but also its ownership as in, who it belongs to. The markers on a cell that indicate its identity are called a cluster of differentiation or CD and they are numbered, based chronologically on their historical discovery. For example a CD4 cell is a T helper cell (a type of white blood cell). If CD4 cells become depleted, as in HIV infection, the body becomes vulnerable to infections. Counting the CD4 cells can then help in determining the severity of the disease. A CD8 receptor is predominantly expressed on natural killer or cytotoxic T cells. In the same fashion, the stem cells carry their own CD markers and on that basis can also be identified and counted as CD34 or CD133 just to name a few. (9)

Besides the clusters of identification, human and animal tissues also have genetically-coded antigens on their surface that help identify self from foreign. These antigens are called Human Leukocyte Antigen (HLA). There are three general groups of HLA; they are HLA-A, HLA-B and HLA-DR. Many different proteins exist within each of these three groups and each of these HLA has a different numerical designation, for example, you may have HLA-A1, while someone else might have HLA-A2. (8)

There is a basic rule in HLA inheritance:

- You have a 25% chance of inheriting all of the same HLA as any one of your siblings,
- You have a 25% chance of not inheriting any of the same HLA, and
- You have a 50% chance of sharing some of your HLA with your siblings.

Each of us therefore has a 1 in 4 chance of being an identical match with our siblings. HLA class antigens are the strongest determinants of rejection of an allogeneic transplant; these loci are therefore important for matching donor and recipient for transplant. If this matching is not conducted carefully the body of the recipient will reject the donor's tissue as foreign and destroy it.

Let us now get back to the battlefield. The first step is the recognition of the enemy. We now know that based on the antigens on the surface of the invading cell, the body's white blood cell (WBC) will recognize and attack any foreign invader whether it is a bacteria, a transplanted cell from someone else or a mutated cancer cell within one's own body. They will all appear as foreign to the WBC soldiers. With this innate ability to recognize a foreign organism or cell, white blood cells, including macrophages, neutrophils, and monocytes, can attack, breakdown and devour parts of or a whole invading organism depending on its size. The recognition system helps the Tcells (T lymphocytes) to usher in other protective and killing cells. In addition a group of cells called natural killer cells are ever ready to recognize and kill cancer cells and cells that are infected with viruses.

Besides these "off the shelf", ready to deploy protector cells, there is another variety of WBC, called B-lymphocytes. These B cells, when presented with a foreign antigen, produce antibodies. Antibodies are proteins that bind to specific antigens and mark them for destruction. In addition, they maintain a memory of this invader in case of a consecutive attack by the same invader. Based on this memory, B-lymphocytes mount a quicker and more robust response each successive time, which probably gave humans an evolutionary advantage. Essentially the T-Lymphocytes are like shotgun shooters who attack all foreign invaders instantly with a wide range approach, whereas the B-Lymphocytes are like snipers who need a little time to steady themselves but take a targeted and calculated aim and hit the precise target.

In addition to cells dispersed throughout the body, our immune system includes several organs. These organs include thymus, spleen, lymph nodes and bone marrow. The bone marrow is where production of all the different types of white blood cells, as well as red blood cells and platelets takes place. It is also the place where the stem cells and precursors of different blood cells reside and work. When needed to defend the body, these marrow precursor cells divide, increase in number and produce white blood cells to be mobilized. They then move into the bloodstream and travel to wherever they are needed. Hopefully the above explanation clarified for you what happens if an unmatched foreign tissue is transplanted in a body.

It is not a unique or infrequent event that our body is attacked by dangerous organisms. These are rather constant threats that are being silently neutralized by our body every waking and sleeping moment of our lives. However, in order to carry out these massive military operations, the body needs a constant supply of the lymphocyte, monocyte, macrophage and other warriors, and that's where the regenerative ability of stem cells comes into play. The stem cells replenish and regenerate the precursor cell pool to maintain our immunity.

# Chapter 4

# STEM CELL

*"There is a principle which is a bar against all information, which is proof against all argument, and which cannot fail to keep man in everlasting ignorance. That principle is condemnation without investigation."*
*~ Herbert Spencer.*

Yeast, fruit fly, mouse and man - what do they have in common? Besides sharing many genes and similar stages of embryonic development, they all start out as a single cell, then depending on the information hidden in the nucleus of that one cell they evolve along very different lines and mature into very different beings. So what is in that one cell?

Let me tell you a love story. Once there was a young rubenesque egg, an incomplete cell who inherited only half the genetic material from its parents (23 chromosomes instead of 46). It held its virgin chromosomes safely in the nucleus. When it reached puberty and the hormones started raging, one day it burst open the doors of the doughy ovary tower and went for a stroll. Covered with a soft fur it was sliding on the shiny peritoneum, when it noticed a pink, fril-lined tunnel leading to an unknown destination. Following its adventurous nature, the egg leaped into the tunnel. There it ran into a large rowdy mob of young sexy sperms swimming in a pool of mucus. One of the sperms caught the egg's attention and it was love at first sight. As the skinny, naked sperm tried to hide its tail, the egg noticed that the sperm also had only half the genetic material (23 chromosomes). Just as this thought came into its mitochondria, the egg heard a voice in the background - "you complete me" and it instantly knew what to do. It ran and embraced the sperm, swallowing it whole, and a Hollywood star was born. In fact that's how every Hollywood star is born.

If you want to know the whole story of this Hollywood star you would need a short lesson in embryology, so here it goes. With the fertilization of the egg by the sperm the two nuclei merge to create a cell complete with 23 <u>pairs</u> or 46 chromosomes, half from each parent including an X from the mother and either an X or a Y from the father. This new cell made by a sperm from the father and the egg from the mother is called the zygote and inside this zygote is the potential to create a complete human being, Hollywood star or not. Mind it though, in nature, only about 1/3 or less of these zygotes ever get implanted in the uterus and even fewer make it to birth. (1)

This is important to remember because until the zygote divides a few times, increasing the number of cells to about 120 (in about 5-6 days' time), it is not ready to implant into the uterus and is still only something of a potential, not nearly a fetus or a baby. Just like the millions of sperms in that mucus pool had the potential to fertilize this egg, only one actually does. The potential of the rest of the million will never come to fruition. I want to seriously stress this point because this juncture in the human development is the main contention over which the embryonic stem cell war is being fought.

So an egg has the potential, but by itself (at least in humans), it cannot produce a fetus, neither can a sperm, though it also has the potential to create a new life, and even though the two gametes fuse to form a zygote at fertilization, in biology there is no specific or defined moment of conception and the process takes place over several hours. Even after the zygote is formed it has only 1/3 or so chance of implanting or progressing to the stage of a fetus. A true biological individual as a unique human is not apparent until much later in the course. In fact, in the first 2 weeks or so, the developing zygote, which is later called a blastocyst, can potentially have several fates. (2)

1 - It may stop progressing and die of genetic or other defects.
2 - It may fail to implant and is discharged.
3 - It may split and become two identical twins or even triplets.
4 - Two simultaneously developing zygotes, fraternal twins, may combine in the uterus, one absorbing the other. The two embryos thus become

one fetus with two distinct genetic complements. (Recent data from The Netherlands suggests that this is not an infrequent occurrence at all). (3)

Do realize that these are not rare possibilities; all of them happen at a fairly high frequency. So you see, at this stage of the first 14 days of development, an identity cannot be applied with certainty to this blastocyst. Assigning personhood at this stage would mean that one person may become two, or two may become one, because:

1 - The blastocyst may divide to become two fetuses, or
2 - Two embryos may fuse to become one fetus.

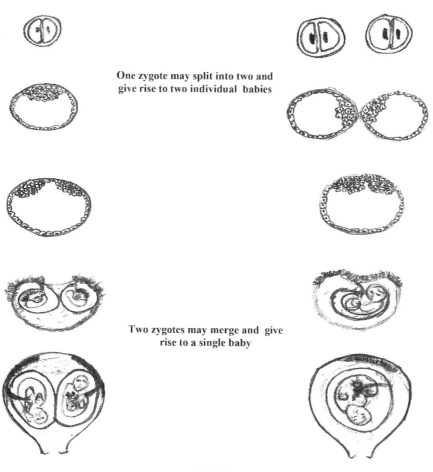

One zygote may split into two and give rise to two individual babies

Two zygotes may merge and give rise to a single baby

(Fig 2)

This discussion becomes even more complex when the fertilization takes place in a petri dish as in case of In-Vitro Fertilization (IVF). Here the zygote may have one other possible fate. It may be used to extract the blastocyst cells for genetic testing or research instead of implanting in a uterus. This eliminates any chance of becoming a fetus.

In IVF, an egg and a sperm are fused to create the zygote that is allowed to progresses to a multi-cell stage, when a vacuole forms inside and moves a cluster of the cells to one side while the rest of the cells line the cavity. The cluster of cells pushed to one side is called the "inner cell mass" that later forms all the cells of the fetus, whereas the cells surrounding the cavity are called the trophoblasts which later become the placenta, cord and the membranes that nourish and protect the developing fetus. At this stage the blastocyst is as big as the dot on the "i" in size. If it were inside the mother it could have implanted in the uterus to start a pregnancy, but if it is in a dish and is never implanted in a uterus it has NO possibility of ever becoming a fetus.

This is the stage in the embryonic development (always before day 14 and always outside the uterus) where the scientists take the cells from the inner cell mass and grow them in cultures to make embryonic stem cell lines. These cells have the potential to make each and every cell type among the more than 200 different varieties of cells in a human body. Therefore these cells are called "pluripotent", with plenty of potential to make any cell. They are not, however, like the 8-16 cells of a dividing zygote before the blastocyst stage which can make all the baby cells plus the placenta, membranes and cord. These earlier cells are hence called "totipotent" since they have total potential to produce every cell required to accomplish a pregnancy.

As the cells in the inner cell mass repeatedly divide and grow in number they start aligning themselves in three flat layers, one on top of the other. This flat mass then curls in a way as if flat-bread curls into a burrito. The inner most layers thus create a tube with openings at both ends. One end is the future mouth and the other the future anus. This entire tube is lined by the inner layer or "endoderm", around it is the middle layer or the "mesoderm", and on the outside is the external layer or the "ectoderm"

The endoderm layer from mouth to anus gives rise to the entire digestive system along with its buds that develop into digestive glands like liver, pancreas, gall bladder, thyroid, as well as lungs. The ectoderm forms the skin with its pigment cells and the entire nervous system including brain, spinal cord and the special sense receptors, like the olfactory smell receptors in the nose, light receptors in the eye or the taste cells in the tongue. The mesoderm which rests in between the inner coil of endoderm and the outer covering of ectoderm makes pretty much all other tissues in the fetus. These include, bone, cartilage, muscles, fat, blood, heart, kidneys, etc.

Therefore, the cells that initially constituted the inner cell mass move in different directions initially into 3 different layers. They then advance into a particular body system, for example, digestive system and later into more specialized organs like stomach or liver cells. As the cells move along in this future direction they become more and more specialized and less and less able to form a wider variety of cell types. In other words they lose their "stemness" as they progress down a certain path. Earlier in development each cell has more potential to give rise to a large variety of cells.

- The zygote cells are totipotent and can create every cell for the baby and the placenta.
- The inner cell mass cells of the blastocyst are pluripotent and can give rise to all the cells of the baby but not of the placenta.
- The cells from any of the 3 layers are multipotent and can give rise essentially to all the cells of the tissues that belong to that particular layer but not necessarily to other layer cells.
- Eventually when the cells are differentiated into their final destiny, for example liver or skin cells, they become unipotent and can only give rise to liver and skin cells.

There is one important caveat and that is, most organs and tissues retain some relatively primitive cells amongst them for future repair and growth. These are called tissue stem cells or adult stem cells. (More on those later).

During embryonic development the cells divide and differentiate into more and more specialized cell types. The stem cells progressively lose their stem characteristics, that is, they lose their ability to specialize or differentiate into several different directions. Each direction previously adopted gets more and more committed to its final cell type. Even though a copy of the entire DNA remains in each and every cell, more and more restricted access to certain DNA areas is granted to the cells down the line of differentiation. Under normal circumstances differentiation is a one-way process; once a cell is terminally differentiated into a specialized cell type, it cannot on its own revert back to a stem cell. This however is a standard scenario and usual scope of things; there are many exceptions and new developments that can be confusing to a casual reader. We will try and clarify those terms and caveats in later chapters.

**What's in a name?**

*That which we call a rose by any other name would smell as sweet*
*~ William Shakespeare*

Before we embark on learning about different types of stem cells, we need to define what a stem cell is. In simple English, a cell from which all or most of an organism's cells stem from is called a "Stem Cell". The quintessential stem cell is a zygote, the first cell that has the potential to give rise to any and all cells required to make a complete human being. The ability of stem cells to differentiate into any kind of cell is called plasticity. As the cells go down the path of development and differentiation into more specialized cells they gradually lose this plasticity or potency.

Based on the source from where they are derived, the stem cells may have different levels of plasticity and can therefore be classified as totipotent, pluripotent, multipotent, or unipotent.

However based on their origin they can be classified as:

| | | |
|---|---|---|
| 1- | Embryonic | From the inner cell mass |
| 2- | Fetal | From the fetal germ cells |
| 3- | Umbilical | From the umbilical cord blood |
| 4- | Adult | From a human baby, birth onwards |
| 5- | Tissue | From the particular tissues of an adult |
| 6- | Induced | From any non-stem cell by induction. |

In general the 1st and 2nd in the above list are generally referred to as embryonic stem cells (ESC), and the 4th and 5th as adult stem cells (ASC), while the 6th one, as induced pluripotent stem cells (iPS cells). (4)

Clearly this nomenclature can be confusing but we will use the generally accepted names and abbreviations.

(ESC) Embryonic stem cells are pluripotent.

(UCSC) Umbilical cord stem cells are multi–pluripotent.

(ASC) Adult Stem cells are multi–pluripotent.

(iPS cells) Induced pluripotent stem cells are pluripotent.

The characteristics of stem cells that separate them from regular body cells are:

- a- Self-renewal: The ability to make more stem cells like itself.
- b- Potency: The potential to differentiate into a variety of cells.
- c- Immortality: The ability to grow almost endlessly.

During the embryonic development, as the cells divide and differentiate into more and more specialized cell types, the stem cells progressively lose the above characteristics. They lose their ability to differentiate into a variety of directions as well as their longevity. Whatever direction each cell adopts, it continues to get more and more committed in that direction of differentiation. This unidirectional increased level of commitment results from the alteration and suppression of many genes which were active during embryonic development as well as changes in the epigenetic messages and codes that lock the cells into their new identity and prevent deviation from their path.

Like an usher at the concert hall, who will let you go towards your seat in your section but not let you jump the barrier and occupy a seat in another balcony, this biological fidelity and commitment is important and prevents such things as a tooth growing in a spot where you had a mole removed. The cells in the vicinity of an injury will only form the particular cells of that organ this saves us the embarrassment of having a toe growing out of our nose after nose-piercing. Though if it did, we could have been spared some unsightly piercings.

I like using the analogy of the education system; we start out with basic high school credentials and later choose science, or business or humanities. If you choose science you later major in a field of engineering or biology and if you go into biology you may end up in medicine, pharmacology, veterinary, dentistry, etc. Selection of medicine can lead you down the path of either clinical or research medicine. If you are inclined towards clinical medicine you will have a variety of options to pick from and specialize in cardiology, surgery, dermatology, etc. If at this stage you want to revert back and become an archeologist, it will not be easy to do so. With a lot of extra coaching, coxing, time, money and effort it may become possible in some cases and so is the case with cells. Once down a path they keep moving towards differentiation in a one way process, or so we thought.

Scientists have now discovered ways to coax these specialized cells using new techniques to help them revert back to their stem cell state; these are called induced pluripotent stem cells or iPS cells. (More on this later).

*We owe almost all our knowledge, not to those who have agreed,*
*but to those who have differed.*
*- Charles Caleb Colton*

# Chapter 5

# HUMAN EMBRYONIC STEM CELLS

Embryonic stem cells are pluripotent cells grown in a culture in the labs that have the potential to give rise to every cell in the human body. Technically, embryonic stem cells do not naturally exist in nature or even in an embryo. These are cells derived from the inner cell mass of the blastocyst stage of a pre-implanted embryo. They can also be derived from the gonad ridge of aborted fetuses.

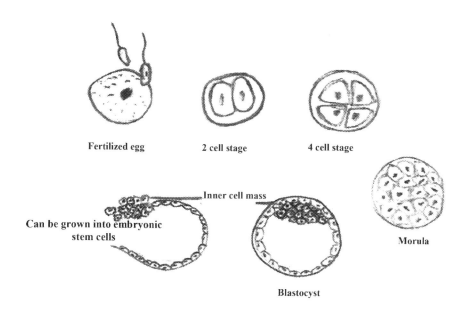

**Source of Embryonic Stem Cells**

(Fig 3)

Because of their high plasticity and nearly unlimited capacity for self-renewal, embryonic stem cell therapies have been proposed for tissue repair in disease or for tissue replacement after injury. Diseases that could potentially be treated by such pluripotent stem cells include a number of blood and immune-disorders, neurologic diseases like multiple sclerosis or Alzheimer's, diabetes, liver or heart failure, blindness, stroke, traumatic brain injuries and spinal cord injuries. They may serve both as a source of cells for transplantation or tissue engineering. (1) Other potential uses of embryonic stem cells include the study of early human development, drug development and the testing and study of genetic diseases.

Most of what we know about embryonic stem cells is information gained from mice and other animal embryo studies. In fact, the first embryonic stem cells were propagated from mice in 1981 by Martin Evans. Later in1998, James Thompson from the University of Wisconsin propagated the first human embryonic stem cells. (2) This was the breakthrough that opened "heaven's door" to so many possibilities and potential cures for a host of devastating diseases. But it also opened "hell's gates" to bitter opposition, name-calling, accusation of playing God, creating monsters, selling fetuses and killing babies.

Experience teaches us that,

- Science is more factual and less emotional;
- Politics is self-promotional and less rational, while
- Media is often barely investigational and highly sensational.

So while scientists present facts and data, politicians continue to promote the core beliefs and views of their support base and the media remains busy sensationalizing both aspects of the debate. That is why you so often hear media stories presented as if next week we will be able to go online, order a new kidney or heart and a bottle of stem cells extracted from some helpless embryo in South Asia just to get rid of our wrinkles and rejuvenate our bodies. Followed by another story where scientists are at the verge of creating mice with human brains. "Experts" sit around contemplating both the horrors and mental capacity of these mice that don't yet exist.

Media representation of scientific breakthroughs; of which stem cell research is a hotbed, generally, is misleading. These stories do usually have a grain of truth over which a mountain of embellishment is heaped, creating a much sensationalized, intriguing, and for most, an "interesting news piece".

Another good example of this is the field of genetics, where practically every month you hear news about how scientists have discovered the gene for autism, for anger, for homosexuality, for leadership or for success. Genetic diseases or personality traits are actually not a matter of one aberration. Often multiple genes, encoded proteins, epigenetic messages and hormonal control, not to mention a number of environmental and developmental factors, are intricately involved in these situations. (3)

Apologies for the digression, my point is that we should take these stories with a grain of salt and do our own due diligence as to what the real truth is. Facts show that embryonic stem cells are the only cells known to us that are truly pluripotent (can give rise to each and every cell type in the body) and immortal (can propagate and divide essentially for ever and ever). As of right now, no cell, even the induced pluripotent stem cells have proven this capability. These facts alone make embryonic stem cells exceptionally unique and full of potential to repair any type of cell in the body, sometime in the future.

This potential, however, comes with a very high price of controversy, because their production results in the destruction of an embryo (more on that in the ethics chapter). Remember embryonic stem cells do not naturally exist in embryos. They are derived from the inner cell mass of the blastocyst. There are other new and novel options to derive embryonic stem cells that do not require fertilization of the egg by a sperm (conception) or even destruction of an embryo. You would think that this ought to limit the objections and controversy, but not so. Alternative techniques either already have, or may potentially in the future, allow the propagation of embryonic stem cells without fertilization or conception. Just like there are more than one ways to skin a cat, so can the blastocysts be created in more ways than one.

# Chapter 6

# ADULT STEM CELLS

During embryonic development, most cells differentiate and become specialized to form a specific organ; some of the cells however maintain their stem cell characteristics. As tissue research progresses, we are finding out that almost all tissues and organs contain a proportion of these stem cells commonly known as adult stem cells.

Potency of these adult stem cells is hotly debated in scientific circles. In general, adult stem cells residing in a specific organ are only multipotent, which means they have a limited range of cell types they can produce. This spectrum is limited only to the organ or system where they belong. For example, hepatic or liver stem cells can form different cell types that constitute the structure of liver, but are not able to form nerve cells. Recent research is, however, showing exceptions to these general rules. When it comes to stem cells derived from bone marrow or fat, this spectrum seems to be much larger than previously believed. Until recently, the prevailing scientific belief was that once differentiated, the final cells must stick to their cellular destiny. Recent research is, however, consistently showing proof otherwise. (1)

Regardless of the level of their potency all these stem cells have the ability to self-renew. Somatic cells like liver, bone, or skin cells divide into two identical daughter cells, the same in nature as the parent itself. Whereas all the stem cells are able to undergo asymmetrical division, whereby at division, they produce one stem cell and one differentiated daughter cell. (2) Another way stem cells self-renew and maintain their pool is by self-replication, thus increasing the number of stem cells, then few of these stem cells go on to differentiate into specialized daughter cells.

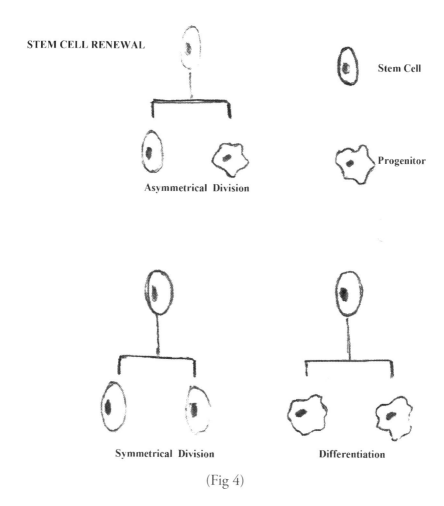

(Fig 4)

Different organs and tissues have different needs for repair and replacement, and they accordingly have a variable number and activity of stem cells. For example, the skin and intestinal mucosa constantly shed cells that need to be replaced. Similarly, blood cells have a short life and require constant regeneration to replace the dead and damaged cells. On the other hand, muscle and bone, under normal circumstances have fewer turnovers and therefore less stem cell activity. (3)

Doctors and researchers knew for centuries that the body has the capacity to heal itself. Nowhere was it more abundantly visible than on the skin. Battle wounds routinely healed and filled in, so it was not surprising that any good observer would have reached the conclusion that the cells in the body have the ability to repair and heal. This belief was also reinforced by observation of regeneration in other creatures in nature. However, it wasn't until the mid-20th century, that researchers came up with the idea of precursor cells. (4)

Various experiments on bone marrow in the 1940s and 1950s provided clues that bone marrow contains cells with an ability to produce a variety of blood components (red cells, white cells, platelets). Their potency however was initially believed to be limited to the formation of blood cells. The regenerative ability of marrow precursor cells was confirmed by experiments in mice whose entire blood and immune-forming system was first killed with radiation and later injected with bone marrow from a healthy mouse. To the researcher's surprise, the cells in the marrow successfully reconstituted the entire blood and immune system in the irradiated mice, with all different cell types. This confirmed that cells in the bone marrow were capable of producing all different types of cells in the blood.

Further studies showed that there was one specific type of precursor cell that was responsible for the reconstruction of the entire blood and immune system. This cell is known as the "hematopoietic stem cell". This stem cell creates daughter cells which serve as precursors or progenitor cells for a variety of blood cells. If you imagine a hematopoietic stem cell to be the grandparent who produces several off springs, each then produce their own distinct family of cells all indirectly belonging to the same blood and immune system family. This way you can easily understand the lineage of the different types of blood cells that can be traced back to one patriarch / matriarch.

Unlike other somatic cells in the body, which normally have a specific function, pancreatic cells produce insulin, thyroid cells produce thyroxin, muscle cells contract, etc., stem cells do not have any such specialized function. They serve as the cells "on-call" for repair and regeneration. In order to fulfil this function they rest and wait for their call, every now and then, self-renewing to maintain their number and strength.

Twenty five years ago when I was in medical school, doctors and scientists believed that all the repairs in the human body are carried out by the tissue specific cells in the injured or affected organ. This was most commonly thought of in the skin and bones. Other organs like the heart and brain, we were taught, were incapable of regeneration and self-repair. The concept of tissue stem cells or a working repair system in the body was nonexistent. Sadly even today, talking to medical students and doctors in different parts of the world, including here at home, I'm shocked to learn that many medical professionals still believe in this obsolete information. Over the last few years, adult stem cells have been identified in almost every tissue of the body including the brain. (5) These adult stem cells are not however, equally prevalent in every tissue. Stem cells in the brain, for instance, have only been identified in the memory center of the hippocampus and the olfactory cells, whereas stem cells are diffusely dispersed in fat, skin and bone marrow.

In any given tissue, stem cells are few and far in between. They form only a small percentage of the total number of cells and they live in a special environment called the "niche". The cells of the niche are suspected to play an important role in keeping stem cells safe, catapulting them into action when needed. This is accomplished with the help of chemical signals and direct cell to cell communication. A variety of signals from neighboring cells and remotely released chemical agents provide a complex control of their division and differentiation.

Based on over half a century of experiments on mice and four decades of bone marrow transplant experience in leukemia patients, doctors and scientists have gained a better understanding of bone marrow stem cells than any other type of stem cells. Our current knowledge tells us that the marrow, not only has hematopoietic stem cells that form blood and immune cells, but also other types of stem cells with a much broader potential.

1 - Mesenchymal stem cells: have the potential to give rise to cells of bone, muscle, fat, cartilage, ligaments, etc. (4)
2 - Endothelial stem cells: can give rise to blood vessels and heart cells.

These stem cells have been identified in the marrow and other tissues (also known as tissue stem cells). They remain difficult to identify and isolate, hiding in niches, they are non-specific in shape and form. The origin of these tissue stem cells is also uncertain. Several hypotheses have been proposed as to their origin, but none has yet been confirmed. Regardless of the origin and despite many similarities, all adult stem cells are not the same. They are abundant, active and energetic in some organs, for example in the liver and bone marrow, but are slow, few and subdued in others, like the heart and brain. As for the origin these may be:

1 - Embryonic cells left by design in each organ during development, for future differentiation.
2 - Circulating embryonic cells that find homes in different tissues at or before birth.
3 - De-differentiating cells inside the tissues which keep them as backup for regenerative activities.

Regardless of their origin, Adult stem cells have tremendous potential and for that, hundreds of promising trials are in progress. Even if only a few of these trials turn out to be successful, many novel therapeutic options may reach clinical use within a decade.

Without a doubt this is great news. However, this is not without challenges, nor can it be assumed to provide definitive solution for every ailment or disease; besides, they also have their limitations. That is why it is not scientifically true or factual when embryonic stem cell opponents allege that "adult stem cells have such great promise; there is no need for embryonic stem cell research". The fact is that adult stem cells do not have as much potency and immortality as the embryonic stem cells do and they are harder to grow. The following are some of the challenges adult stem cells pose.

Disadvantages of adult stem cells:

1 - The do not usually form cells outside their tissue type.
2 - They are rare; most tissues have only a small percentage of adult stem cells.
3 - Extracting adult stem cells from a donor usually requires invasive procedures.
4 - They neither divide very often, nor for very long (have early senescence).

5 - It is nearly impossible to grow large numbers of adult stem cells in the laboratory.

6 - In case of hereditary genetic diseases, adult stem cells from the patient cannot be used for treatment because they also carry the genetic defect.

7 - Allogeneic adult stem cells; those from another adult, carry the risk of rejection.

Not all adult stem cells have the same potential; hence they pose different intensities of the above challenges. Some adult stem cells are easy to extract such as hematopoietic stem cells from the marrow, but much harder to grow outside the body. Others, such as mesenchymal stem cells from fat need extraction using a mini liposuction, but grow rather well in the laboratory culture environments. Yet other tissue cells require a biopsy. Easy accessibility of the fat and marrow is part of the reason why most of the adult stem cell trials involve the use of mesenchymal stem cells. The number, health and activity of the adult stem cells in a tissue determine its regenerative capacity. In the chapter on keeping your stem cells healthy, I will discuss the do's and don'ts of keeping your own stem cell population in optimal condition and higher number.

Advantages of adult stem cells:

The biggest social advantage of adult stem cells use is the lack of controversy involved with embryonic stem cells. This does not however rule out governmental and regulatory challenges.

Besides this social advantage, adult stem cells also have a number of biological advantages:

1 - They are present and available in all human adults.

2 - Their autologous (patient's own) stem cell use avoids rejection.

3 - Adult stem cells differentiate well into mature organ or tissue cells instead of getting stuck at some level of immaturity; which embryonic stem cells sometimes do.

4 - Adult stem cells have a relatively lower risk of cancer formation, when compared with embryonic stem cells.

5 - More recently, varieties of adult stem cells have been discovered that offer higher differentiation potential.

# Chapter 7

# UMBLICAL CORD STEM CELLS

*He who joyfully marches to music in rank and file has already*
*earned my contempt. He has been given a large brain by*
*mistake, since for him the spinal cord would suffice.*
*-Albert Einstein*

For centuries, the placenta and cord have received ceremonial handling by many cultures around the world. Some local tribes in Nigeria and Ghana treat it as the twin of the baby and give placenta full burial rites under a tree. Burial of the placenta is a common tradition throughout Africa and parts of Asia. New Zealand Maori, Native Americans and native people of Hawaii also bury the placenta and cord. Other traditions dry it and use it for medicinal purposes. Traditional Chinese medicine considered the placenta a powerful and sacred medicine – an organ 'full of life force'. It was recommended for consumption by the new mother to support healing. Chinese medical texts from 1578 list the umbilical cord tissue and blood as a medical product.

This medicinal value was also acknowledged in western countries. Historic records show that in 1994, Britain banned the practice of collecting placentas in hospitals after learning that 360 tons of it was annually being bought and shipped by French pharmaceutical firms. These French companies were using the placentas in their cosmetic products. Encapsulated dried placental tissue was also sold for treatment in Europe and the Americas leading upto the 20th century... It makes you wonder if our ancestors knew something about the healing properties of this tissue, which we are only learning now.

During pregnancy the umbilical cord keeps the baby connected to the placenta. Later at birth it seperates from the baby however, some blood remains in the cord and placenta which can easily be collected without any risk to either the mother or the baby. Once discarded as waste, it is now in wide demand for its stem cell content. Umbilical Cord Stem Cells (UCSC) are collected from the afterbirth and preserved for later use. Some off shore facilities use these cells for the treatment of a variety of diseases. However, such treatments, without FDA approval, can not be performed legally in any USA jurisdiction.

It is interesting to note that the FDA restricts the allogeneic stem cell use by doctors in any form. However, since 1984, the allogeneic umbilical cord derived cells have been used in transplants for leukemia and other blood diseases in the USA with FDA approval. They already have a great safety and decent efficacy record. The same method of preparation and administration however, if used to help anyother disease in a patient, may land the physician in jail. The early experimental treatments with umbilical cord blood in cancer patients were also anecdotal, without clinical trials, and were entirely based on the courage and competence of innovative physicians. just like the ones who performed the first heart transplant or kidney transplant.

The umbilical cord blood is rich in hematopoietic stem cells and other primitive cells. These cells are considered adult because they no longer have embryonic features and in their nature are more like adult cells though much younger in chronological age. Given their youth and immaturity they have better replicative and regenerative capacity than other cells. The nature of their immaturity also seems to give them an advantage known as immune privilege. This means they are too immature to have firm identification symbols and thus are less likely to be rejected. This has been observed in patients with leukemia who had umbilical cord blood transplant rather than an allogeneic bone marrow transplant from a donor. In fact mesenchymal stem cells (MSC) from umbilical cord blood have been shown to prevent or reduce the severity of graft versus host disease. Cord blood therefore offers a useful alternative to bone marrow transplants for some patients.

This immune privileged nature of umbilical blood cells is quite significant. This characteristic of the fetal blood has been noted in clinical settings under the name "maternal microchimerism". During normal pregnancies some cells from the baby escape the placenta and enter the mother's circulation. Although genetically foreign to the mother, they do not cause any reaction; in fact they contribute to the normal healing and repair process in the mother's body. Therefore, we have long time clinical experience of the natural introduction of these umbilical cord blood cells into an unmatched recipient (mother) without any reaction or side effects, rather therapeutic benefit.

The placenta is a better source of stem cells as it contains approximately ten times more stem cells than the cord blood. One drawback of using umbilical cord blood for an adult patient is the lack of sufficient quantity of stem cells in a single cord. A transplant containing too few hematopoietic stem cells (HSCs) may fail. This has been experimentally overcome, very recently, with the discovery of a molecule UM171 at the University of Montreal. UM171 can increase the number of UCBC ten times in the lab. This new discovery may overcome the quantity problem.

A number of researchers are also pursuing safety and efficacy trials on umbilical cord stem cells in humans for therapeutic use other than blood cancers. (1, 2) These indications include:

Use of cord blood stem cells after brain injury, (3) type 1 diabetes, (4) treatments following stroke, (5, 6) Cerebral Palsy (7) and hearing loss (8). Their use in cardiac disease has also shown promising results including the ability to migrate to injured cardiac tissue, improve local vascular functions and blood flow as well as improve overall heart functions. (9) A new kind of cord blood stem cell has now been identified which displays both embryonic and hematopoietic characteristics and is multipotent. This type of cell demonstrates embryonic cell markers as well as leukocyte antigen CD45. (10)

Another placental source of stem cells that is increasing in popularity is found in the tissue of the umbilical cord and placenta known as "Wharton's jelly". This is a rich source of Mesenchymal stem cells (MSC). Tissue of the umbilical cord can yield between 21 million and 500 million MSC which have the potential to differentiate into bone, cartilage and connective tissue cells. (11) They are also effective in mediating inflammatory response in the body. (12) There are also some reports of an improvement in Type 1 diabetes when treated with infusion of autologous cord blood. (13) Additionally, multipotent stem cells are also found in amniotic fluid. These stem cells are very active, expand extensively with ease and do not produce tumors. Amniotic stem cells are multipotent and can differentiate into a variety of cells. (14)

The research is ongoing, the studies and trials are progressing, and media and journals are filled with new information daily with sometimes encouraging and at other times discouraging news. When the dust settles we will know what actually works and will be part of our future medical care and what will be relegated to the annals of history. But all indications are that MSC are inching ahead in the game.

I feel confident that we are approaching an era where instead of hearing the news of a discovery we will more often be hearing the use of a discovery. Based on available information it won't be wrong to predict that within the next few years therapeutic products derived from umbilical cord blood would be available in the market for clinical use. Grown and enhanced, under good manufacturing practice protocols they will be patented, priced, and marketed for use.

# Chapter 8

# INDUCED PLURIPOTENT STEM CELLS (iPSc)

*"There are many ways of going forward, only one way
of standing still." ~ Franklin D. Roosevelt*

In the preceding chapter we learned the origins, characteristics and limitations of different varieties of stem cells - embryonic, adult and from the umbilical cord. All these different types have their advantages and disadvantages, benefits and limitations. Some are easy to use, but difficult to obtain. Others have ethical, legal, or logistical problems. In order to move the research forward, necessity indicated the need for a pluripotent cell that had the potential of an embryonic cell but no religious, ethical or legal baggage -- a cell that will be more "self" so as not to be rejected by the patient, but not as hard to extract as an adult stem cell and not so sensitive to require a human egg for its production.

As you know, necessity is the mother of invention. Well! Invention's mother got pregnant with possibilities, and a brilliant scientist from Japan, Sanaya Yamanaka, started testing his Nobel Prize winning theory. He knew that all cells have the entire DNA code in them from embryo to adult and that the change in the activity of the DNA at different stages of development results from the turning on and off of certain genes. He proposed that cells would go back from adult to embryonic state if you could reverse this cascade of gene-tuning sequence.

His hypothesis was first tested in mice using manufactured viruses to insert certain factors into the DNA of a mouse's cells. This procedure was able to reprogram mouse cells back to embryonic state. After further refinement of the technique he found that it requires just four factors to achieve this retrograde march of adult cells towards embryonic state. (1)

First announced in 2006, the news of these "induced pluripotent stem cells" (iPSc) sounded too good to be true. However, within a year, human induced pluripotent stem cells (iPS cells) were presented, not only by Yamanaka's team but also by James Thompson's team (with the use of a slightly different combination of factors). (2)

The process of developing induced pluripotent stem cells (iPSc) is relatively simple and can easily be learned. Within a few years, most laboratories had become able to generate their own induced pluripotent cell lines. The iPS cells have now become a common and easily accessible source for stem cell research. This brought in a breakthrough that overcame the funding and the ethical restrictions, catapulting the field into a new, bigger and brighter space. The massive benefits of the induced pluripotent stem cell technology are:

1 - No human egg or sperm is required.
2 - No embryo is either created or destroyed.
3 - The cells come from the patient, so have the same genetic makeup and therefore carry no risk of rejection.
4 - Cells are easy and non-invasive to extract, and can easily be taken from the skin or connective tissue.
5 - They have theoretically the pluripotency of embryonic stem cells so they can be developed into a wide variety of cell lines.

In fact, since their discovery iPS cells have been generated from many adult somatic cells by converting them into the embryonic state, and then marching them step-by-step in many different directions to produce pancreas, liver, brain, heart, and many other cell types. On top of that, cells from diseased persons have also been converted into iPS cells, and then differentiated into specific diseased tissue cells in order to:

1 - Understand and study the defect and mechanisms of that disease.

2 - Test treatment options on those cells, providing more realistic results as to how the human diseased cells will likely respond to the therapy.

This is often referred to as the "disease in a dish," model. This application is one of the supreme benefits of iPS cells that is already showing great promise, and has the potential to not only help discover new drugs, but do it faster and cheaper than ever before. In the last five years, many laboratories have already succeeded in generating iPS cell lines from patients of ALS, Diabetes, Parkinson's, and hundreds of other rare, and common diseases.

The ability to watch these cells grow and differentiate into the diseased cells is expected to unfold and reveal critical steps where things go wrong or where correction ought to be attempted. This promises to allow the understanding of each disease process, and hence strategies to cure them. The breakthrough that Yamanaka and his team created opened the floodgates of new innovative ideas about how to study disease, test treatments and reprogram cells.

One exceptionally fascinating idea is that if a mature cell can be reprogrammed all the way back to embryonic state, and then programmed again, for example into a pancreatic cell, would it not be possible to program it directly into a pancreatic cell, without first going to the embryonic state? This implies a short cut, instead of a long march back to embryo and a new forward march in a different direction. Scientists, therefore, explored programing that cut to the chase and went from one cell directly to the desired cell of another kind.

Historically, one such example had already been provided by Dr.Harold Weintraub. 10 years before the advent of iPS cells, Dr.Weintraub described a myoblast determination gene (MYOD) that alone could reprogram fibroblasts (one of the commonest supporting cell in the body) into myoblast (muscle precursor cell). Just this one factor can change mature cells like fibroblasts into muscle cells. This is called direct reprogramming, (3) which are becoming more prevalent by the day.

Advances since the initial iPS cells development have allowed discontinuation of the virus use to induce the DNA change. Messenger RNAs or even safer molecules can now be used to create the iPS cells, thus removing a major objection to their use; risk of accidental introduction of a virus in the patient with the iPS cell. (4).

As promising as iPS cells sound and look, they are not completely free of problems either. For one, the safety of treatment derived from iPS cells has not been proven. There have been concerns that programming can possibly cause a mutation in the genes, and that the differentiated cells derived from iPS cells are not exactly like the differentiated cells derived from human embryonic stem cells. Another factor with iPS cells is the cost and the time it takes to produce and validate their cell lines. However, both of these are expected to decrease with newer technology and techniques. One recently raised concern is based on the observation that sometimes these reprogrammed iPS cells revert back to their original adult state without any warning and for yet unknown reasons.

Additionally, people who are bound to find an issue with stem cell research have raised objection to the iPS cell research as well. This time their issue is with the theoretical likelihood, if at all, that someday in the future it may become possible that iPS cell technology may lead to a way that may provide a remote possibility of an unlikely successful human cloning. Like I said, some people will find objection to anything that threatens to shake the quagmire of obsolescent, stagnant, status quo thinking that they are embedded in.

The real worry, however, is that since the iPS cells are pluripotent, like the embryonic stem cells, by definition they can form teratomas, or other tumors, or may be cancers. At this stage we just don't know. However, neither with human embryonic stem cells (hESC) nor with iPS cells, there is intent to use them in their pluripotent state. It is clear that for clinical use these cells will have to be nudged and coaxed into differentiated precursors of the desired cell type before they are injected into a patient. This is expected to significantly reduce both the risk of cancer as well as undesirable differentiation. Definite lineage differentiation prior to injection in the patient will allow for more controlled development of the desired target cells.

Additional advancements are now moving towards direct differentiation, straight from one cell to the other. A Stanford group recently skipped the intermediate embryonic like stage altogether and converted mouse skin cells directly into neurons. (5) Reprograming is not limited to mice. Human skin cells have also been converted into blood cells through direct reprogramming, bypassing the iPS cell stage. (6)

The following are some of the preclinical advancements in the field of iPS cells that will give you some idea of how rapidly we are moving in the direction of advanced regenerative medicine. Scientists have generated iPS-based cells for many different organs, allowing them to study the causes and potential treatments for a range of diseases.

In the eye these include diseases which can cause blindness such as age-related macular degeneration. (7) Other animal models are for spinal cord injuries, where iPS cells differentiated into functional nerve cells, are being studied for cell-replacement therapy. (8) iPS cell technology also provides a new platform for understanding heart disease. This offers new tools for evaluating drug treatments and the possibility of restoring heart muscle damaged from ischemia. (9, 10) Similarly, iPS derived kidney cells are helping to better understand kidney disease and likely treatment options. (11) iPS-derived liver and pancreas cells have also been developed to study the underlying causes of liver and pancreatic illnesses as well as to evaluate potential drugs to treat them. The pancreatic cells have been shown to secrete insulin when transplanted in animal models. (12, 13) Researchers have also transformed human iPS cells into insulin-producing cells that, when transplanted into mice with Type I diabetes, help control blood sugar.

For the musculoskeletal system diseases human iPS cells have been reprogrammed into bone and cartilage cells which in the future will be likely candidates for the treatment of damaged cartilage or osteoporosis. (14, 15)

> *"There are two ways to be fooled. One is to believe what isn't true; the other is to refuse to believe what is true." – Søren Kierkegaard.*

The question that has repeatedly been asked but never satisfactorily been answered is... Can iPS cells replace hESC? (human embryonic stem cells). Despite the claims by pro-life groups that they do, the jury is still out. What we should consider is the fact that it has been nearly a decade since the development of iPS cells, but their safety and complete clinical potential remains unclear. I believe all of the above; embryonic, fetal, adult and induced pluripotent stem cells have a role to play in teaching us the steps of the development of a normal as well as a diseased tissue, from the common progenitor cells of the embryo to the terminal diseased tissue in a patient. It will be premature and unwise to give up any one of these avenues of research and exploration. Who knows what secrets to human development they may be waiting to teach us, or what method of human rescue from illness they may hold.

# Chapter 9

# ETHICS AND STEM CELLS

*Our human compassion binds us one to the other - not in pity*
*or patronizingly, but as human beings who have learnt how to*
*turn our common suffering into hope for the future.*
*~ Nelson Mandela*

As you read this, a war continues to rage over the issue of the rights of a fertilized egg, an embryo, and millions who await the advancement of stem cell research into definitive therapies for their ailments. Should a fertilized egg be given full rights as a human being? At what stage does life begin? When should a fetus be granted personhood? Should there be different laws governing therapeutic vs. reproductive cloning?

Governments and groups are suing scientists for unethical behavior. There are attorneys in court rooms representing unborn fetuses, fighting to declare some two cell organism, a human and religious groups are predicting this to be the end of times. It is not a matter of who is right and who is wrong. It is a matter of what is morally and ethically acceptable for humanity and at what cost.

Here I want to examine the nature of ethical and moral reality for yesterday, today and tomorrow. You may know some or all of the following examples but let us refresh our memories anyway.

1 - On 15th October 1872, Mrs. Virginia Minor, a native born, white citizen of the United States from state of Missouri, presented at the registrar of voters, to register for the upcoming November presidential

election. She was refused because she was not male as ordained by the State of Missouri: "Every male citizen of the United States shall be entitled to vote." Ms. Minor sued the state and the case was decided by the Supreme Court which delivered the following opinion: The court reaffirmed in a unanimous decision upholding that the constitution of the United States does not guarantee women the right to vote.

"For nearly ninety years the people have acted upon the idea that the Constitution, when it conferred citizenship, did not necessarily confer the right of suffrage. ............ no argument as to the woman's need of suffrage can be considered." Chief Justice Waite - Minor vs Happerdett; Supreme Court of the United States; 88 U.S. 162; 21, Wall. 162.

2 - In 1958, Mr. Richard Loving, a white man, married one Mildred Jeter, a black woman, in the District of Columbia. They later relocated to Caroline County, Virginia where they were charged with violating Virginia's ban on interracial marriages, sentenced one year in jail, and barred from living in Virginia for 25 years. The Supreme Court justices read the following decision. Similar decisions were handed down by several other states against interracial marriages. (1)

"Almighty God created the races white, black, yellow, malay and red, and he placed them on separate continents. And, but for the interference with his arrangement, there would be no cause for such marriage. The fact that he separated the races shows that he did not intend for the races to mix" - Chief Justice Warren; Loving vs. Virginia (No. 395); Court decision 1958.

3 - August 1982, one Michael Hardwick was given a citation for public drinking by an Atlanta police officer, Keith Torick. Days later, while visiting Mr. Hardwick's house, Officer Torick allegedly entered the house using an invalid and already recalled warrant. He searched the house without permission and found and arrested Hardwick in a compromising position in bed with a same sex partner. Hardwick sued the state for violation of privacy and his constitutional rights. The case finally reached the Supreme Court. (2)

Justices Byron White and Warren Burger of the US Supreme Court wrote the decision in the Bowers vs. Hardwick, 478 U.S. 186 (1986) that emphasized historical negative attitudes toward homosexuals, quoting Sir William Blackstone's characterization of homosexuality as "a crime not fit to be named." Justice Warren Burger concluded, "To hold that the act of homosexuality is somehow protected as a fundamental right would be to cast aside millennia of moral teaching."

Similar decisions were handed down on many occasions and by several states against same sex marriages. Nearly all of those decisions have since been overturned. Inter-racial marriages and voting rights for women are now legal in all states. Same sex marriages after last month's supreme court decision are now legal in all 50 states. (3)

But you should not be surprised to hear that there are many who believe that these unfair and prejudicial decisions were actually correct and should not have been overturned. Unlike religious commandments, social laws are dynamic. Ethics relating to specific actions are not set in stone, and the definition of morality changes in the context of the discussion and the age of time. Nowhere is it more acutely evidenced than in science and medicine.

Laws reflecting the beliefs of the time are nothing new. Interracial marriage was still illegal in Alabama in 2000. In Arkansas there still exists a law instated in the 1800s according to which a husband is allowed to beat his wife, once a month. In Massachusetts it is deemed illegal for a woman to be on top during intercourse. In Iowa it is illegal for a man with a mustache to kiss a woman in public. In Oregon talking dirty while having sex is illegal. In Vermont a wife needs the husband's permission to wear false teeth. In Kentucky a woman cannot remarry the same man more than three times. In Honolulu Hawaii, it is illegal to sing loudly after sunset. In Florida it's illegal to fart in a public place after 6 pm on a Thursday. Good times! In Good ol' US of A.

What about rest of the world?

In Saudi Arabia it is illegal for a woman to drive a car. In Dubai extramarital sex is against the law and carries a jail sentences for over a year. In Samoa it is illegal to forget your wife's birthday. Divorce is illegal in the Philippines. In

Singapore selling or chewing gum as well as spitting are illegal and can result in an arrest. In Thailand it is illegal to step on money.

Oh! So you think it only happens in the east? Read on.

Ancient Greeks prohibited Athenians from marrying foreigners. (4) In Greece police are allowed to arrest anyone suspected of having HIV, and to have them evicted from their homes. In Victoria, Australia it is illegal to change a light bulb unless you're a licensed electrician. In Britain it is an act of treason to place a postage stamp bearing the monarch's head upside down. In France it is illegal to marry a dead person. In Switzerland it is illegal to flush a toilet after 10 pm. If you have stopped laughing, let us talk some sense.

Just because a belief was accepted by most as a norm yesterday or is today does not make it "normal" (whatever that is) or right. During World War II, Japanese Americans were compelled to move into relocation camps by Civilian Restrictive Order No. 1, 8 Fed. Reg. 982.5. Every legal American citizen of Japanese descent on the West Coast was rounded up, just to make sure they didn't "turn on us". One Japanese-American Fred Korematsu evaded internment and sued the US government. The case went all the way to the Supreme Court, which ruled 6-3 in favor of the internment of the Japanese American and Korematsu was convicted of internment evasion. *Korematsu v. United States*, 323 U.S. 214 (1944). (6)

Carrie Buck was a 17 year old girl in 1927, living in Indiana with her foster parents, the Dobbs. According to historic records she was raped by Dobb's nephew and got pregnant. Using the state's feeble-minded law, she was institutionalized and, pursuant to the Indiana law, ordered to be sterilized. The State determined that the Buck family line was "defective". Despite Carrie's appeal, a number of "experts" testified in favor of her sterilization and Justice Oliver Wendell Holmes of the Supreme Court handed the ruling in an 8-1 decision in favor of sterilization. (7) Not only Carrie, but her younger sister was also sterilized, to prevent the spread of "feeble-mindedness" in the Buck family.

Tens of thousands of people, mostly minorities, underwent compulsory sterilization during the last century. This was Eugenics plain and simple; an effort to improve the genetic features of human populations through selective breeding and sterilization. Eugenics was practiced in the United States many years before similar eugenics programs were adopted in the Nazi Germany. In fact many Nazi German leaders alleged US programs to be the inspiration for their own actions. (8)

In the USA eugenics was considered a method of preserving and improving the dominant groups of the population. This was based on the belief that Nordic, Germanic and Anglo-Saxon people are genetically superior. They achieved their goal by providing support of strict immigration and anti-miscegenation laws, and forcible sterilization of the poor, disabled and perceived "immoral".

Even today, eugenics is still officially permitted in the United States. In Californian prisons alone, close to 150 women were sterilized between 2006 and 2010. And as recently as 2012, a Massachusetts judge ordered a pregnant schizophrenic woman to have an abortion and be sterilized to prevent the spread of her faulty genes. That's right, terminate her pregnancy and sterilize her because she is mentally ill. The order was stopped, after the poor woman appealed. (9)

It's not always the governments behaving badly; no apple grove is free of bad apples. The horridly sick example of that is the Tuskegee syphilis experiment. This was the infamous clinical study from 1932 to 1972 conducted by the U.S. Public Health Service with the stated goal to study the natural progression of untreated syphilis. Until that time there was no need for an informed consent, ethics approval or oversight by an institutional review board in matters of medical research.

Even though syphilis was not a disease limited to the black race, investigators enrolled a total of 600 all black subjects in the study. 399 of those men had previously contracted syphilis, and 201 were without the disease. None of the men were ever told that they had syphilis. According to the Centers for Disease Control (CDC), the men were told they were being treated for "bad blood"; a non-specific term for various illnesses. Eight years into the forty-year long study, penicillin became available and by 1947 it was firmly established as the cure for syphilis. However, none of the participants in the study were treated with penicillin. Not only were they not treated, scientists even prevented participants from accessing other syphilis treatment programs in the area. The study continued until 1972, when a whistleblower leaked the real proceedings to the press and the resulting public outrage caused the termination of the study. (10) By the time of its termination, 28 men had already died of syphilis and an additional 100 from its complications. 40 of the participants' wives had contracted the infection and at least 19 children of these participants acquired syphilis at birth.

In the post World War II period, following the revelation of atrocities of the holocaust and medical abuses by the Nazi's, changes in international law, and formulation of the Nuremberg Code were enacted to protect the rights of research subjects. However, none of this impacted the continuation of the Tuskegee syphilis experiment. What is worse, the study was not a secret, reports and data sets were published in professional journals throughout its duration without any objections raised by the medical community. The study was supported at all levels by the Public Health Service. Even after it became a public disgrace and termination was ordered, Dr. John Heller, then Director of the Public Health Service's Division of Venereal Disease, gave the following statement," For the most part, doctors and civil servants simply did their jobs, some merely followed orders, others worked for the glory of science." (11)

The Center for Disease Control (CDC) was in control of the study at that time and reaffirmed the need to continue the study until completion, which meant the death of all participating subjects and performance of their autopsies. The CDC's position was strengthened by both the National Medical Association (of African-American physicians) and the American Medical Association (AMA).

I will let you make up your own mind, as to how a small group of misguided professionals, public officials, and scientists can enforce what they call ethics, and get fairly broad support for their actions in this day and age. I mean this was going on as we were doing heart transplants, making computers, landing on the moon, and ironically building Holocaust memorials. While in our own backyard the Tuskegee study was inching towards 40 years of moral and ethical indignity and ignominy.

I believe we should think twice when we are deciding for others or on behalf of others ...how our decisions will impact them and how these decisions will be judged tomorrow, when even today, right here in my gut I feel it to be absolutely wrong.

Recall from previous chapters how an IVF embryo is generated. Just like in nature, only a fraction of IVF blastocysts (less than 40 %) ever implant into the uterine wall and progress to a baby. Therefore, as a precaution, fertility clinics prepare several spare embryos in order to achieve a successful pregnancy, (12)

The leftover embryos can later be used to create another pregnancy. However, if the parents do not want any more children, they may give permission to donate these embryos to another couple. If no decision is made then the leftover embryos are stored away in freezers only to be discarded later as bio-waste. It would seem logical that these extra embryos should be adopted by other infertile couples but in reality this is not a common scenario. Most couples want their own genetic offspring and many parents of the leftover embryos don't like the idea of someone else raising their biological offspring.

Whatever the reason may be, the historical reality is that the majority of the extra embryos from IVF clinics are destroyed without much noise, fear of God's wrath or legal repercussions. However, if from any of these extra embryos, destined for the trash bin, cells are taken to be grown for research (embryonic stem cells) then all hell breaks loose.

Sounds crazy? It does to me too, but it is the honest truth. The standard practice of dealing with hundreds of thousands of extra embryos from IVF fertility clinics is to discard them, because they are no longer needed by their biological parents, have not been permitted for adoption, and are restricted for use in federally-funded research.

Despite what politicians may tell you, except for the biological parents, no one has the legal right to decide the fate of these embryos in limbo. However, if with the parents' permission the scientists take the cells from the inner cell mass, technically those cells were not capable of forming a fetus anyway because they were never going to be implanted in a uterus.

The reason underlying the controversy is that, in order to propagate the embryonic stem cells from the inner cell mass of the 5 to 8-day-old pre-implantation embryo, it has to be sacrificed. The ethical concern in this context arises based on the belief as to when does human life begin? There is clearly no "scientific answer" to this question. In fact there is also no "right answer". I will, however, offer a rational answer, which other countries have also used to decide their own ethical laws relating to embryonic stem cells. Though I know it will not satisfy many beliefs, here is how I think and I am sure many readers will disagree, so with all due respect.

In everyday clinical medicine, following all accepted ethical guidelines and with the permission of the family, there comes a time when a person is declared dead and all life-support is discontinued (13) despite the fact that the body still feels warm, the chest is still heaving with breath and you can still feel the pulse. But by all scientific standards the person is brain dead, and we accept them to be without life.

At this point if the family gives permission, life support is discontinued, the deceased's organs are harvested and tissues maybe collected for the purpose of research. Full dignity of the deceased and respect and feelings of the loved ones are honored. However, some family members challenge this declaration of death and the patient remains on life support, brain dead for weeks or months, in exceptional cases for years. In the loved one's mind, there remains the "potential" that the patient will survive, when in reality that is not possible.

The other end of the spectrum of life is the embryonic development. Scientists and doctors cannot pinpoint when life begins. They can, however, tell us when the heart starts beating (around 12 weeks) or when the neurons start firing (after the first trimester). In fact, we even know when the first heart and brain cells start to form and differentiate. Before that point, the embryo is a lump of cells secreting fluid with no differentiated heart, liver or brain cells. The neural cleft, which is the earliest indication of the formation of the nervous system, occurs around day 14. This might be the reason why in some religions, it is believed that the soul enters the fetus on day 14.

*The energy of the mind is the essence of life. - Aristotle.*

Around day 14 is also the time when the embryo implants into the uterus. Implantation is a crucial step in the development of the fetus because in nature less than one-third of all embryos successfully implant and develop into a fetus. (14) If not implanted, the embryo does not thrive and is lost in menstrual blood.

Based on the above information, beliefs of some religions, laws of several western countries and a few legal precedents, I myself, and many others tend to believe that life begins sometime after implantation around day 14 of embryonic development and at the formation of the neural cleft. Of course, I have no authority or absolute knowledge of this fact but neither does anyone else.

Despite the common assumption that doctors can tell you when human life begins, every doctor I have ever asked this question reverts back to his/her religion for answers. (15) Their answers span from:

1 - Before conception, at the stage of egg and sperm.
2 - Conception, the actual fertilization of egg and sperm.
3 - Development of neural cleft.
4 - Beginning of heartbeat.
5 - Independent survival or survival outside the mother.

There is no way to prove or disprove any of the above assumptions, or to convince someone one way or the other. Though one thing is clear, potential does not equal product. Every child has the potential and right to drive a car, but we don't hand them the keys until a specific age and skill level is reached. Similarly, if I try to sell you a dozen apple seeds and charge you for a dozen apples, you may want to send me for therapy or jail.

This argument is also supported by the fact that the grief, mourning and burial proceedings are directly proportional to the stage of the development of the fetus. The mother is not expected to face the same grief for the loss of a 1 month old pregnancy as she is for the loss of a 7 month old pregnancy. Neither is the family expected to hold a funeral for a 1 month aborted fetus as they are for a still birth. With this line of thinking, if contraception is avoided with the idea that every egg and sperm has the potential for conception and life and therefore should be preserved, then masturbation and menstruation should be followed by funerals.

There are not enough pages in this or any book that would settle this argument. So I urge you to remember that the embryonic stem cells we are discussing here are not EVER derived from a pregnancy. They are extracted with the permission of the parents from leftover IVF embryos that are less than 14 days old, sitting in some fertility clinic freezer not intended for implantation in a uterus. If not used for research or for embryonic stem cell lines, these embryos will either stay frozen and become unviable or eventually be rendered unusable and discarded as bio-waste.

The question you should be asking yourself is how any of these alternatives are better, than giving these embryos some dignified humane purpose? In fact, embryonic stem cell extraction allows these embryos, destined to be disposed off, an amazing potential. It is the potential to give life, not only to one fetus, but to hundreds or thousands of people whose lives may be saved with the use of their cells. In some ways, this is not dissimilar to harvesting organs from an imminently diseased donor, with the permission of the guardian or loved ones.

I wish my passion was contagious, but after having debates with the opponents of the embryonic stem cell research, I know it to be wishful thinking. So I would let you be the judge. I understand the argument that in order to draw the inner cell mass the embryo is destroyed and I do agree with the idea that no one should be allowed to create a human embryo with the intention to destroy it, regardless of the extent of research gain, but when you have embryos that would be literally thrown down the drain, then I fail to understand the objection to their use for relieving the suffering of many many humans. To me it is not different than preserving the organs of someone who will soon be buried or cremated but their tissues can still be used to save lives. (16)

However, for those who shout bloody murder when you mention the embryonic stem cell research, they close their ears and their minds before you can get to any rational point. They follow the same doctrine as the people who claimed that allowing blood transfusion interferes with the will of God, who argued that using pig valves to fix human hearts is dehumanizing, and they are the same who claimed IVF to be an abomination, a sign of impending doom. They predicted a future of mechanized human reproduction and female exploitation.

During the debates over IVF in 1978, at the birth of the first test tube baby in England, they professed that test tube babies will soon be in the black market. Now more than a quarter century has passed and we haven't seen any Armageddon, human baby factories or a black market selling test tube babies.

What we did see is tens of thousands of childless couples give birth to their own children who are being raised in loving homes.

Some people with this same philosophy and dogmatic thinking are once again professing that embryonic stem cell research is the harbinger of human organ factories and dungeons of human clones. They akin creating embryonic stem cell lines to armies of cloned soldiers and towns full of deformed human hybrids. They paint a grotesque picture of the scientists and doctors who are propelling the stem cell science forward, comparing them to devil worshippers and Frankenstein creators.

I wonder if these folks have an active imagination or they completely miss the facts of science. Do they blindly follow some misinformed zealot or a misdirected politician? The bigotry is that over centuries, the people behind the anti-vaccination, anti-transfusion, anti-IVF, anti-transplant campaigns, have themselves, and their loved ones, taken full advantage of these life-saving procedures in the years that followed; after spending droves of money and energy to deny the same right to so many others, until their absurd assertions were proven wrong beyond every reasonable doubt.

I have no doubt that they will again one day benefit from the progress and advancement of the stem cells revolution. However, their ignorance may have denied the same benefit to many who don't have the luxury of time to wait till the debate is over.

> *"All truths are easy to understand once they are discovered;*
> *the point is to discover them." ~ Galileo*

I have two comments.

One that in IVF procedures a large number of extra embryos are produced and routinely damaged, discarded, destroyed, or if you prefer, killed. So how come no one is stopping the IVF procedures?

Second, many couples opt to have their IVF embryos genetically tested for abnormalities prior to implantation. This procedure is called pre-implantation genetic diagnosis (PGD or PIGD) and in this procedure a cell from either the

8 cell stage or the blastocyst stage embryo is removed and tested for genetic abnormalities. Clinics that offer PGD often provide it for sex selection as in "family balancing" where a couple with children of one sex desires a child of the other sex. PGD can potentially be used to select an embryo without genetic disorders, to match an HLA type in order to produce a tissue or organ donor, or to have a baby with less cancer predisposition. (17)

In any case embryos that test positive for "undesirable traits" are discarded. So why are pro-life advocates not stopping this? How come it is legal? This is genetic screening, to have a baby of your desired sex, or of an HLA type that can be used as a tissue donor for your own or one of your children's transplant treatment.

Where is the ethics in this? Is it OK to first discover that the potential life in the embryo is defective or of the wrong HLA type before we destroy it? But it is not OK that the embryo slated for destruction is used to advance science or to help find cures for human suffering?

I find the rigid, irrational, dogmatic opposition to embryonic and other stem cell research to be more anti-life than it is purported to be pro-life. For all the lives that could have been saved if the stem cell research and treatments were allowed to proceed unhindered, the blame should be on the shoulders of those who prevented it. They essentially allowed thousands of innocent patients to suffer and die while they placarded, bull-horned and mass-emailed their resistance to medical advancement. I wonder if there was a law that prevented everyone from availing a cure in the future that they prevented someone else from recieving in the past; would there be such resistance to stem cell cures?

> *"I would rather make mistakes in kindness and compassion than work miracles in unkindness and hardness." ~ Mother Teresa,*

In my clinical practice I come across all kinds of people. As a physician, I treat all of them with the same care and dignity, regardless of their color, sex, race, sexual orientation, age, and political or religious views. However, over the last 20 years of my practice I have sadly encountered families who have very strong views about certain aspects of treatment and research, but only until either themselves or one of their loved ones need that care and then you can hear them back paddle to rationalize the acceptance of that option.

There is this one story that I remember rather clearly because it involved multiple prolonged arguments with the daughter of a local priest in East Texas. She was a patient of mine who I was treating for diabetes related neuropathy. I clearly recall what a vocal activist and vehement opponent of stem cells she was. This was the year 2004; she did not even understand the difference between adult and embryonic stem cells, all she understood was that no one should be allowed to make "stem cells". I had many conversations with her attempting to explain the science but instead of listening she was always preparing in her mind what she was going to say next so I could never get through to her. In short, she made me her pet project and frequently brought in anti-stem cell propaganda material.

Some of the material she presented to me over the years included religious arguments against stem cell research that were prepared by her father. In 2010, one day this patient came into my office with her father who had developed Parkinson's disease over the years and had stopped responding to traditional treatment. He had been deteriorating progressively when they came in for consultation. I discussed all the possible treatment options but knowing their views about stem cell, left out the potential option of experimental stem cell trial. Ironically, as we approached the end of the consultation she asked me if I could refer him to someone who is practicing the latest treatment for Parkinson's disease using stem cells. I told them of the recent success some institutions had had with the use of fetal tissue. (18) Unfortunately I was not aware of any active trial at that time. I guided them to the website ClinicalTrials.gov to keep an eye, and when one does become available they may be able to take advantage of that. After being declined as a suitable subject for fetal stem cell trial, her father is now undergoing aggressive rehabilitation and pharmacological optimization but the prognosis remains grim.

I vividly remember the expressions on the daughter's face, how hard it must have been for her to ask that question, but I realize that when we have no hope or we see our loved ones suffering, our motivations are different, our compassion is intense and our rationalization changes direction. I believe, we, as humans should have the same compassion for others who are suffering without alternatives and everyday searching for a ray of hope; we should not deny them their right to recovery or relief. We should do very deep soul-searching before we get on a bandwagon, without knowing its direction, understanding its mission, its agenda, or knowing the motivations of the person who is in the driver's seat. Keep in mind that down the road you or a loved one may be the next victim this bandwagon will run over.

> *"Compassion is the basis of morality."*
> *-Arthur Schopenhauer*

I urge the government to make laws to prevent development of any embryo with the intent of destruction; ban human reproductive cloning; restrict the use of embryonic stem cells derived from embryos developed with the intent of destruction. (19) But please do not discard hundreds of thousands of embryos but deny the possibility to use them for research which may help us find relief for suffering. For goodness's sake, don't deny millions of humans the hope and chance to have a disease-free, pain-free life, while you pack these embryos in a red biohazard bag to be burned.

# Chapter 10

# VIRGIN BIRTH TO HUMAN CLONING

Virgin birth used to be a major fascination of our ancient ancestors. From the 6000-year-old history of the Sumerian culture, recorded on clay tablets, to Greek and Roman mythology, to the monothestic books of God, you will find stories and references to virgin birth everywhere. If there was anything like Hollywood during the Roman Empire, I'm sure they would have made movies about virgin birth, just like Hollywood churns out movies about cloning (*Boys from Brazil, Multiplicity, Jurassic Park, Star Wars Episode II: Attack of the Clones, the Expanded Universe or the Clone Wars…...*).

Reproductive cloning is generally the focus of these science-fiction movies that attract awards and accolades. In real life however, cloning has drawn a lot of skepticism, controversy and criticism from all types of organizations. The more useful and purposeful part of the cloning spectrum for medical use is therapeutic cloning, which does not get nearly as much press. (1, 2) This however, is one area where technology is likely to be used in a positive manner for the benefit of society. Who would have thought that virgin birth and human clones could be discussed together in one conversation about embryonic stem cells? Stranger things have happened in the battlefield that is stem cells. Let me explain.

As the controversy and the ensuing restrictions and bans on embryonic stem cell research became heated, some scientists started leaving the country for nations with better research opportunities and more liberal laws. Others limited their research to non-embryonic stem cells while the rest started working on alternate ways to get around the roadblocks by using the frozen embryos.

The goal of embryonic stem cell research is not to destroy human life, rather to save millions of lives. The effort of the scientists, therefore, moved to exploring ways to develop embryonic or embryonic-like pluripotent stem cells from blastocysts without fertilization or even without the need of a blastocyst. Necessity is the mother of invention, and so the maternal instincts kicked in once again. The following developed as theoretical and practical possibilities for propagating embryonic stem cells without using the fertilized egg or IVF embryos.

PARTHENOGENESIS:

Parthenogenesis is a Greek word meaning virgin birth, though parthenogenesis widely occurs in other living creatures, it has never been documented in humans. (3) In the lab, however, it is a different story. A human egg can be artificially activated without any involvement of the sperm and coaxed into developing at least upto the blastocyst stage. It doesn't progress much past that level of development, so no risk of a virgin birth there.

As you know, from the blastocyst stage, the inner cell mass can be taken and grown into embryonic stem cells. However, in case of parthenogenesis these cells can only be female, because there is no male or Y chromosome involved. Scientists agree that it is not possible today, given the current reach of technology and science, to progress this into a fetus. Theoretically, and maybe one day practically, parthenogenesis could have the potential to result in pregnancy and birth. This begs the question; if embryonic stem cells are drawn from parthenogenesis induced embryo would there be any less objection to this process? It also reaises a valid notion that the egg alone has potential for creating life, which will give egg the same status as an embryo.

HUMAN CLONING:

According to ancient alien theorists, from the text found on the 6000 year old Sumerian clay tablets from the civilization of Mesopotamia (modern day Iraq) comes the very first documented creation myth. According to this creation story, humans were cloned to perform labor by an advance alien race called Anunnaki (of the royal blood). (4)

Sumerian language experts who have interpreted these texts give an elaborate account of the origin of human species in their writings. (5) According to these ancient translated documents, the story goes something like this....

At first, two sacred substances named "Teima" (things that retain memory, assumed to be DNA or genes) and "Sill" (thing that can only be gathered from Anunnaki males assumed to be sperm) were gathered from the bodies of the Anunnaki. Then the Teima and Sill were mixed in a clean bottle with an ape-woman ovum. That is, the ape-woman ovum was fertilized with the sperm of the Anunnaki. The fertilized egg was then moved from the clean bottle to a mold and grown there for a fixed period of time. After that, the fertilized egg was implanted into the womb of the Birth Goddess, that is, the womb of an Anunnaki woman who became the mother.

The whole story that the Anunnaki created the new humans, that is, earthlings, as a hybrid between Anunnaki and the ape-man from earth, is allegedly well described in Sumerian ancient documents. Looking at the description of the procedure, it appears someone is documenting a laboratory reproduction of a test-tube baby (IVF). What happened next is described in translated texts of the ancient alien believers, as follows....

The Birth Goddess watched over it. A scientist of the Anunnaki counted the months. The fateful tenth month came, but the time for the womb to open passed (this is to say, the birth didn't begin even though it was overdue). Then Ninharsag "covered his head with a cloth, and opened the womb using tools, and took a fetus out. Ninharsag rose the "new born being "up high, and shouted while shaking with joy. "I have created! My hands have made it!"

An earthling was hence born in the image of its creator; a hybrid between the Anunnaki and the ape-man, and deliverd apparently by a Caesarean section. The hypothesis of human cloning by aliens is based on the premise that Anunnaki scientists created earthling clones to labor in their place. According to this description, the lower ranks of the Anunnaki, who were assigned to hard labor in the earth's gold mines, rebelled against the leader, so the leaders of a higher rank, came to Earth and held a meeting. In that meeting the scientists suggested "There is our Birth Goddess, so let her create a slave worker. Let that being be yoked, let that being bear the toil of the Gods". Translations of the ancient Sumerian documents allege that these circumstances produced the first human being; an earthling. The man was called "Lulu" in Sumerian which means "mixed one". Once Anunnaki had created a complete human, they mass-produced them for labor using the cloning techniques.

I do not expect you to believe any part of this myth. I certainly do not want to add yet another fairy tale over which believing cultures can fight and kill. (6) Considering how strange this story is, it does remind me of Mark Twain.

*"Truth is stranger than fiction." ~ Mark Twain*

Let us then discuss the truth about cloning. Genetically identical copies of a biological entity are known as clones. In nature, some plants and single-cell organisms like bacteria can produce genetically identical off springs or clones through asexual reproduction. In asexual reproduction, a new individual is generated from a copy of a single parent cell. Identical twins, in humans and other mammals, are also examples of clones in nature. These twins are produced when an early embryo splits, creating two or more embryos that carry DNA identical to each other but different from either parents.

Cloning plants by growing a new sapling from another plant's cutting, has been practiced for hundreds, perhaps thousands of years. In science the very first account of animal cloning is from 1938 when Hans Spemann published nuclear transfer experiments in which he transferred one cell's nucleus into an egg without a nucleus, providing the basis for subsequent cloning experiments. Research continued in a variety of species and in 1962 John Gurdon cloned a South African frog using the nucleus of an adult intestinal cell. Though he didn't himself use the term cloning, scientifically that's what it was. Then the race was on. Karl Illmensee cloned mice, (7) and several other animal clones were attempted but what made animal cloning popular was "Dolly the sheep". Dolly was the first vertebrate to be cloned from the udder cell of an adult sheep, using the Somatic Cell Nuclear Transfer (SCNT). On July 5th 1996, Dolly was born as a result of the cloning technique developed by Ian Wilmut and Keith Campbell of the Roslin Institute in Scotland.

Culmination of this experiment put an end to the dogma that adult cells cannot be reprogrammed. (8)

Though Dolly was born relatively healthy and bore three healthy lambs (conceived by natural mating), she developed early arthritis and died after 6 1/2 years. The expected life span of her species of sheep is 12 years. Multiple other animals have successfully been cloned since then, including dogs, cattle, monkeys and a cat, aptly known as "copycat", but apparently the technique is not well perfected and all clones have had health problems.

In 2002, a Bahamas based company named Clonaid, with philosophical ties to the Raëlian sect (which sees cloning as the first step in achieving immortality), claimed that a cloned human baby named "Eve" was born somewhere outside the USA. Media coverage of the claim sparked serious criticism and ethical debate that lasted more than a year. USA Attorneys tried to force the company into producing the baby in court. However, Dr. Boisselier, the CEO of the company did not present either the mother or child. Legal attempts to expose the claim failed due to jurisdictional technicalities. In 2003, Clonaid, announced the birth of a second "cloned" baby, this time in Europe, again, without any tangible proof. (9)

Despite such publicised claims and rumors there is no evidence that a human has ever been cloned. Based on what we know, as of right now, science is not capable of consummating this fascination. Additionally, no legitimate scientist is interested in or supportive of human cloning. There has never been any known objection to the ban on human reproductive cloning. The thorny issue is the medically and scientifically beneficial therapeutic cloning.

Most people relate the term cloning only to the creation of identical human beings. This is not true. There are several different types of artificial cloning:

**Gene cloning:** Is the most common type of cloning. It produces copies or segments of DNA and is the technology used to clone bacteria which in turn produce a number of desired proteins for human use. The procedure consists of inserting a gene from one organism, often referred to as "foreign DNA," into the genetic material of a carrier, called a vector. (10) Examples of vectors include bacteria, yeast cells, or viruses. After the gene is inserted, the vector is placed in laboratory conditions that prompt it to multiply, resulting in the gene being copied many times over. An example is the production of human insulin using this DNA recombinant technique, where the human insulin gene is inserted into either bacteria or yeast whose clones replicate while producing insulin.

**Therapeutic cloning:** Is the technique where a somatic (body cell) nucleus is inserted in an enucleated egg (egg whose nucleus has been removed), or a somatic cell's nucleus is transferred (SCNT). This egg is then artificially stimulated, developing into a blastocyst. The embryonic stem cells derived from this blastocyst's inner cell mass are genetically identical; a clone of the borrowed nucleus. (11) This process is called Somatic Cell Nuclear Transfer (SCNT) which can lead to either therapeutic or reproductive cloning depending on whether the blastocyst is used for its inner cell mass or is implanted in a uterus. The therapeutic cloning produces embryonic stem cells for experiments aimed at creating tissues, replacing cells of diseased organs or for other kinds of research.

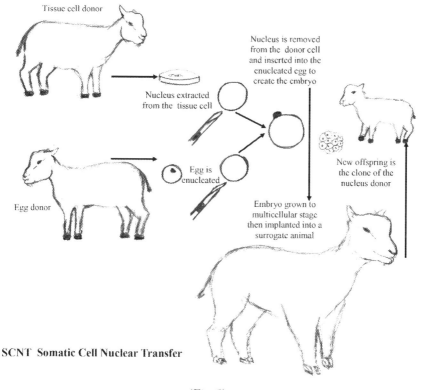

**SCNT  Somatic Cell Nuclear Transfer**

(Fig 5)

Success in therapeutic cloning only requires the development of the embryo for up to 8 days. This does not translate into similar success in reproductive cloning which requires development of up to day 14 for implantation and further progression to a fetus. Years of primate studies especially in monkeys that utilized somatic cell nuclear transfer have never successfully produced monkey clones. It is believed that this is also the case with humans. Furthermore, the comparative fragility of human cells as noted during studies is a significant factor that would likely prevent the development of clones any time in the near future.

**Reproductive cloning:** Is the process which produces copies of whole animals. It has successfully been performed in many species but not in humans because it is illegal in every country that has cloning laws. In reproductive cloning, researchers remove a mature body cell, (somatic cell) for example from skin of an animal that they wish to copy or clone. They then transfer the DNA of the donor animal's nucleus into an egg cell, or oocyte, that has had its own nucleus removed. Researchers can add the DNA from the donor cell to the empty egg in two different ways. In the first method, they remove the nucleus of the somatic cell with a needle and inject it into the empty egg. In the second approach, they use an electrical current to fuse the entire somatic cell with the empty egg. In both processes, the egg is allowed to develop into an early-stage embryo in a test-tube and is then implanted into the womb of an adult animal just like the IVF in humans.

This is the critical step of differentiation between therapeutic and reproductive cloning. In therapeutic cloning no implantation is intended or performed and so there is no chance of a pregnancy. Whereas in reproductive cloning, the ultimate goal is for the adult female to give birth to an animal that has the same genetic make-up as the donor. This young animal is referred to as a clone. Reproductive cloning may require the use of a surrogate mother to allow development of the cloned embryo, as was the case for the most famous, cloned organism, Dolly the sheep.

# Chapter 11

# HYBRIDS, CYBRIDS AND CHIMERAS

*"Do not fear to be eccentric in opinion, for every opinion now accepted was once eccentric." ~ Bertrand Russell*

I was in high school when I first got my hands on a copy of the 9th century BC "Iliad" by Homer. There I read the stories that are claimed to be the source of alternate versions in many of the ancient world's religions. The stories were fascinating and sometimes scary. I remember one in particular where the handsome Bellerophon, riding his Pegasus, kills the fire-breathing monster. I will share some of it with you here.

Sisyphus was the legendary king of Corinth who had a brave grandson named Bellerophon, the son of Sea God Poseidon. Bellerophon was irresistibly handsome, so handsome that King Proetus's wife Antea lusted after him and tried to seduce him. When he showed no interest in her advances she was humiliated and accused him of attempted rape. Being a guest in the king's house, the king had to spare his life, instead he sent him on the quest to kill the beast which had the head of a lion, serpent for its tail and a body that had a goat head sticking out of its back. This 3 headed creature breathed deadly fire and was known as"Chimera". Chimera belonged to a family of monsters; her father was the giant Typhon and her mother, half-serpent Echidna. Her brothers were Hydra, the multi-headed water snake with the uncanny ability to regrow heads and Orthrus the multi-headed dog, guardian of hell.

Bellerophon not only had beauty, he also had brains, so he convinced the flying horse, Pegasus, to help him with this task. On this Pegasus he flew above the Chimera, avoiding her breath of flames and used his ingenious lead arrowhead with which he shot the neck of the creature. The lead melted from the heat of Chimera's own fire and blocked her throat, thus killing the monster.

The Chimera was killed by the hero; however, to this day its replicas and images adorn museums around the world. A mosaic depicting Bellerophon killing the Chimera is displayed at the Rhodes archaeological museum. An ear-stud, with Pegasus and Chimera on the band adorns the Louvre, Paris, and a Chimera from Karkemishhang is at the Museum of Anatolian Civilizations, to name just a few. (1)

So what does this mythical character has to do with stem cells? Well! The fact that multiple genetic identities within one creature is not a new concept. Creatures like Chimera, Sphinx, and mermaids have lived in the fascination of humans for ages. (2) It is possible that others who read Iliad or Odyssey at a young impressionable age have some leftover fears that still scare them at night and they are afraid that if scientists are allowed to do experiments on stem cells and use animal eggs and human genes, the monsters of their nightmares will come alive.

What they don't realize is that they may have just learned about it, but these experiments have been ongoing for decades and no monsters have jumped out of the test tubes as yet. (3) Quite the contrary, a massive number of discoveries and technical knowhow that has been helping develop remedies and discover cures came out of these research endeavors. The reasons why such "unnatural" combinations are produced by scientists include the opportunity to study cell development, and study the genetic basis of certain diseases including cancer, Alzheimer's, etc. and an opportunity to try drugs or therapies on these cells or animals that have human DNA. In this way the research data is likely to be more predictive and closely related than data from animal models alone. This mixing of materials additionally provides a way to conduct experiments which cannot be ethically or legally performed on humans. So you rightfully ask who has a problem with this research. Again, the answer is, ill-informed people who complain and criticize first and learn later, or just believe everything they see on TV, without understanding, exploring or having full knowledge of the subject. I will break it down here for a better understanding.

The mixing of cells can either be a natural or artificial phenomenon. (4) Natural, when a chimera is the result of a spontaneous process, and artificial, when produced from the manipulation and mixing of cells or embryos in a petri dish. An example of naturally occurring chimeras includes twin embryos that fuse in the uterus either at the zygote or early embryo stage. As a result the so called "vanishing twins," can result, where the surviving baby carries the cells from the absorbed twin and is thus a chimera of the two genetic individuals, one from each embryo. (5)

If this fusion happens at a later stage of development it can result in conjoined twins with various levels of complexity, extra limbs, shared organs, joined bodies, etc. New research is showing that chimeras are lot more prevalent in nature than previously believed. Apparently many of us start as a pair of twins only to fuse at some stage and are born with only few minor remnants of the lost sibling, which remain undetectable and don't usually cause any problems. (6) The exceptions happen when a significant number of a person's cells come from the lost twin and they essentially have two different genetic identities within one body. In this case they have some cells with one DNA and other cells with another DNA. This has, on occasions, caused difficulties in matching for organ transplantation, and criminal investigations involving DNA testing and maternity / paternity testing. All of these at some point or another have made for interesting storylines in TV dramas.

Unlike Chimeras, "hybrid" these days is a rather innocuous term, as in hybrid batteries or hybrid cars. Just like hybrid vehicles espouse two or more power sources (gas and electric), hybrid animals or plants are organisms with two genetic sources. A hybrid plant is a cross between two different plant varieties. They are not uncommon. It happens in nature all the time, when two different species cross-pollinate. In agriculture however, hybrids are carefully developed to either take advantage of the strengths or overcome the weaknesses of a single species. They may be designed for disease resistance, ideal size, or enhanced color. Most modern plants are hybrids of some kind. (7)

Common examples of plant hybrids are: limequat, a hybrid of a lime and a kumquat; loganberry, a hybrid between a raspberry and a blackberry; peppermint, a hybrid between spearmint and a water mint, and tangelo, a hybrid of a Mandarin orange and a pomelo or a grapefruit.

Animal hybridization also occurs naturally in the wild from cross breeding between different species, no differently than what dog breeders allow in kennels or veterinary clinics. Examples of animal hybrids are: mule, a cross of a female horse and a male donkey; zonkey, a cross of a zebra and a donkey; zorse, a zebra and horse cross; geep, a sheep and goat hybrid; liger, the offspring of a male lion and a female tiger, whereas tigon is the offspring of a male tiger and a female lion.

By definition, cross-breeding in humans also produces hybrid babies with features from both parents. However, in the lab, when a hybrid is created, it may be by using a mouse embryo and genetic material from a human to create cell lines that have a hybrid origin and these cells are used to study the development of disease. Don't panic, these are not mice with human heads, just cells removed at the stage of early embryo to develop cell lines for study of their performance and activity.

Once you understand hybrids, "cybrids" are relatively easier to understand, you only have to recall and remember three things: (8)

1 - At the time of fertilization the egg is a complete cell with a nucleus and large amount of cytoplasm with all its organelles including mitochondria but half the number of chromosomes.

2 - The sperm is pretty much just the nuclear material, packed tight in a membrane with nearly no cytoplasm or organelles around it.

3 - All of the genetic material in a cell is normally in the nucleus with one minor exception: there is some primitive DNA inside the mitochondria so when the sperm and egg fuse, 99.9% DNA comes from the two nuclei (sperm & egg) but 0.1% DNA comes from mitochondria, in this case the egg mitochondria, since the sperm does not have any.

Recall now, that in the Somatic Cell Nuclear Transfer (SCNT) technique the nucleus of an egg is removed and the nucleus from another cell is inserted in its place. (9) The egg is then jolted electrically to start dividing and becomes a zygote. In this scenario the resulting offspring will have the full nuclear DNA from the donor's parents plus the cytoplasmic DNA from the mitochondria of the egg and therefore is a cytoplasmic-nuclear hybrid, or cybrid.

This is also practiced in IVF (in vitro fertilization) clinics, in couples where the cause of infertility is a defect in the biological mother's egg. To overcome this, an egg is taken from an unrelated human donor. From this egg the nucleus is removed and replaced by the nucleus of the prospective mother's egg. This corrected egg is then fertilized with the sperm of the father. The resulting baby is essentially the genetic offspring of three parents. Scientifically speaking, this baby has three sources of DNA, two from the nuclear DNA of the father and the mother and the third from the egg donor's cytoplasm and is therefore a cybrid. This procedure has recently been made legal in UK.

Today there are many such cybrids walking this earth. Cybrids are also created in the lab. Since human eggs are hard to come by, researchers sometimes use animal eggs, remove their nucleus and replace it with human DNA. (10) The resulting zygotes are not capable of growing into mice with human arms and legs since they do not progress very far in development, but far enough to give cell-lines with human genetic material for study.

Despite what some people may think about this line of research, understanding this clone, hybrid and cybrid technology has helped the scientists a lot in creating appropriate animal modes to study human diseases and come up with meaningful treatments. Once you understand the science and its limits, it is not difficult to understand the reasons behind doing some of these experiments that sound so "weird". Human genes, cells, tissues and their functions are very complex and we need ingenious ways to study and understand them. In order to do that we need such models and avoid experimentation on human subjects.

# Chapter 12

# HEALING IS AN INSIDE JOB

*In science it often happens that scientists say, 'You know that's a really good argument; my position is mistaken,' and then they would actually change their minds and you never hear that old view from them again. They really do. It doesn't happen as often as it should, because scientists are human and change is sometimes painful. But it happens every day. I cannot recall the last time something like that happened in politics or religion. - Carl Sagan*

From time immemorial, the ability of the human body to heal itself has been observed and documented in every known culture. The keen observers of their time noted how the battle wounds closed and broken bones healed. They learned that providing a sick body rest, supportive care, a good diet and a general, healthy environment, allowed it to do its job of self-healing. Though care of the sick has evolved by a large magnitude over the millennia, not much has changed when it comes to relying on the body's ability to self-heal. To this day, no matter what the therapeutic method may be, the eventual reliance is on the restorative and regenerative capacity of the body to accomplish healing. Our external treatments may kill the offending agents that cause infection, limit the damage caused by the disease or help keep the wound clean, but the body repairs and heals the damage from inside.

Though observed and appreciated for ages, this process of healing was quite misunderstood, until recently. The traditional belief stated that the mature cells in any tissue divide to repair the damaged organs. Some organs were believed not to have this healing or repair capability; organs like the heart and brain were believed to be doomed to slow damage and deterioration over time.

Though the concept of stem cells has been known for over a century, it was not in the terms of today's understanding. Marrow was believed to be the only source of stem cells and the potency of these stem cells was believed to be limited to the production of just blood cells (red, white and platelets). There was no appreciation of the regenerative capability of these marrow cells and no recognition of the varieties of stem cells that exist not just in the marrow but essentially in all other organs.

Since the beginning of the 21st century, a number of discoveries in medical and embryological science have proved many long-held dogmas inaccurate one after another. The cumulative effect of this has been the recognition of a naturally-occurring healing system in the human body causing a paradigm shift in medical thinking, these discoveries were as follows:

1 - The discovery of adult stem cells in practically every organ and tissue, including the brain and heart with the ability to not only divide, self-renew and differentiate into local tissue cells, but also with an innate ability to make other types of cells.

2 - The scientific proof that the bone marrow not only contains hematopoietic stem cells which produce blood cells, but also a variety of other stem cells with enormous ability to make numerous types of cells in the body. These marrow stem cells include Mesenchymal Stem Cells (MSC) Very Small Embryonic like Stem Cells (VSELs) Multipotent Adult Progenitor cells (MAPC) and Blastomere like Stem Cells (BLSC).

3 - Recognition of the steps involved in the complex task of self-healing which include:

    a- Signals released from injured tissue into the blood beckon distant stem cells from the marrow towards the injury site,

    b- Stem cells are released from their bone marrow niches in response to the injury signals (eg. Granulocyte Colony Stimulating Factor GCSF),

    c- Stem cells move into the blood stream and start trafficking towards the injury site, and d- Stem cells from the blood, flow into the injured area and migrate into the damaged site along a chemical gradient of chemokines released from injured cells.

Discovery of the complex steps involved in how these newly arrived stem cells create a home in the injured tossue and accomplish repair, further clarified their role and the overall picture of the healing system, as follows:

1 - They secrete growth factors and other chemicals which stimulate vascular repair and retard inflammatory damage,
2 - They stimulate the local stem cell population to spring into action and divide,
3 - They fuse with the damaged cells and somehow help repair and preserve them, and
4 - In small numbers they themselves differentiate into the injured tissue cells causing direct regeneration, as opposed to indirect repair from the above 3 steps.

All of the above steps in the natural stem cell healing system have now been scientifically studied and validated. When combined and looked at as a comprehensive map, it shows the bigger picture of the natural healing and repair in the human body.

We don't completely understand every step of this process yet, neither have we identified every chemical molecule and factor involved therein. We may not know the reason why these stem cells fuse with the injured cells, or the reason for the paucity of their terminal differentiation into the damaged tissue cells. However, what we do know is that health is a balance between the body's ability to repair and replace the damaged cells at the same rate as they are being damaged or destroyed. An imbalance such as absent or retarded repair results in persistent illness or slow healing of wounds and fractures. Too aggressive or too rapid a regeneration of cells, on the other hand, may result in proud flesh, hypertrophic scars or even tumors.

Disease or illness is the result of some kind of insult or damage to the body. The reason it persists or spreads, however, is either due to the rapid rate of tissue destruction or retarded rate of body's repair system too slow to maintain a healthy balance. Old age, smoking, immune suppression, etc. can all compromise the healing mechanisms. In these scenarios, medical therapies attempt to re-introduce balance by either helping to eradicate or retard the offending agents. (For example use of antibiotics to kill bacteria or the use of disease modifying agents to limit collateral damage, such as anti-inflammatory medications).

The new paradigm shift in medicine, however, dictates that in the future there will be a new approach to treating illness. An approach focused on boosting the natural healing system of the body or infusing the body with a large number of healing cells from an external source. This is not much different than transfusing blood after a trauma or blood loss. In fact blood transfusion is a good metaphor to eplain this. We know that the body continuously produces new blood cells to replace the old and dying cells. However, if there is a sudden or drastic blood loss, the production speed of the marrow cannot keep up with the loss. In this case, stopping the blood loss with pressure, suturing, or surgery alone will not be sufficient; the lost cells must also be replenished.

Providing the body with iron, vitamin C, protein and fluid will allow the body to manufacture new cells for long term management. The acute replenishment, however, would have to be accomplished by transfusing matching blood. This is an allogeneic transfusion (from another person). In contract, for pre-planned surgeries, patients often donate their own blood a few weeks prior to surgery which is kept in cold storage. The patient in the meantime synthesizes new blood to replace the donated blood while the donated blood is later used to replace the blood lost during surgery. This is an autologous blood transfusion (from the patient's own body).

A similar process happens in all other tissues. For instance, in the case of pneumonia, bacteria invade the lung tissue, the immune system fights with the invaders resulting in debris of dead bacteria and dead fighter cells as well as collateral damage to surrounding cells from the inflammatory response. When the immune system is strong and the invading bacteria not aggressive, the body will overcome the attack and recover over time. That is how some patients used to survive lung infections before the advent of antibiotics. However, if the bacteria is strong, aggressive and replicates at a rate faster than the body can replenish and repair itself, it will overwhelm the healing and fighting system and overtake the body, causing wide-spread destruction and eventual death. This is where medical treatment steps in, adding antibiotics that kill the bacteria, shift the odds of winning in favor of the body. Realize however, that if the doctor incorrectly chooses an antibiotic that doesn't kill the bacteria, or if the bacteria has evolved and become resistant to certain antibiotic (super bug or drug resistant bacteria), it will continue to wreak havoc.

In both scenarios and in many others like these, the eventual healing and recovery remains the forte of the body that repairs and regenerates. In the future, the recovery from infection, injury and any other disease process (internal or external) is likely to involve not only challenging the invader or the disease-inciting agent but also boosting the defender or the home team of stem cells. This is likely to be accomplished by either agents that stimulate and support the release and movement of stem cells, or external substitution with supplementary stem cells to repair the damage regardless of the agent that caused it. We are already noticing the correlation between low stem cell count and a number of diseases. Studies have shown that hypertension, arthritis, lupus, kidney failure and migraines are all associated with low levels of stem cells.

PROOF IS IN THE GFP PUDDING:

Earlier in the chapter you read claims about stem cells, which heal, repair and restore. Naturally the question comes to mind as to how did we come to know any of this actually happens? Another more piercing question is, how come with all the medical advances and technologies, no one, until recently, had either known about this natural healing system or how it works? And last, but not the least, is the question; does any of this discussed here, has scientific peer reviewed evidence or support.

To the last question the answer is an emphatic - Yes! You can check hundreds of references at the end of this book, but we will discuss it in detail in later chapters. The answer to the other two questions is as follows. The existence of an object, entity, or process, remains a mystery until the day the appropriate tool is discovered which can reveal the secret of their existence.

Galaxies and stars, billions of light years away existed even before our earth came into existence, but their presence was undiscovered by humans until we developed telescopes powerful enough to peek that far into our universe. Similarly, bacteria and viruses, atoms and their nuclei, have all been there as long as there has been life on earth, but we humans were oblivious to it all until we developed microscopes and electron microscopes to discover their existence. The tool and agent that helped disclose the actions and functions of stem cells and the secrets of regeneration came in the form of a much smaller and simpler molecule, though important enough to win the 2008 Nobel Prize for Chemistry.

Green Fluorescent Protein (GFP) is a spontaneously fluorescent protein extracted from a jelly fish (1). The unique thing about GFP is that it is a protein. So like all other proteins, it is coded by a DNA sequence, hence it can be extracted and inserted into the DNA of any other cell using a simple technique of genetic-engineering. Once the Green Fluorescent Protein (GFP) gene is inserted into a cell's DNA, the cell and all its progeny will start producing the fluorescent protein. This will allow it to become easily visible due to luminescence. This ingenious use of the GFP discovery has allowed the study of cells and what they do in the body by following the fluorescent trail. In this way the fate of a single cell can be traced and recorded in an animal showing how many times it divides, what its daughter cells look like, where they go and what they do. (2)

The simple genetic engineering technique above has now been used for many years in research. The genetic code for a protein (a chain of several 3-base amino acid codons results in the synthesis of a protein), can be incorporated into any DNA molecule which, in turn, will start coding for the protein in that cell. This is the method used by pharmaceutical and chemical companies to produce protein-based hormones or chemicals. Researchers use this method to manipulate and create experimental models in cell lines and animals for testing and exploration of disease or treatments.

This is a simple but important concept to understand the stem cell studies described here. Once the Green Fluorescent Protein (GFP) gene has been inserted into a stem cell, all cells derived from it will produce the fluorescent protein and that fluorescence can be detected everywhere those cells go. Using this technique, a researcher produces GFP positive stem cells and injects them into normal and injured mice and other experimental animals. By tracing the fate of these GFP positive cells they are able to show that stem cells do migrate to the site of injury. There is hardly any organ they are not able to go to, if that organ is injured. They automatically reach the injury site, replicate and transform into other cells. Researchers have also noted that uninjured animals or uninjured side of the body do not attract these cells or "home" them in their tissue. Once in the injured tissue, the stem cells differentiate into the local tissue type of that organ. This has been confirmed by the later histological examination of the injured tissue. (3)

In a model of a liver-injured mouse, the injected Green Fluorescent Protein (GFP) positive stem cells localized to the liver and morphed into liver cells, (4) while in a muscle injury model they migrated to the injured leg muscle and transformed into muscle cells but did not home into the leg muscles on the uninjured side. This reinforces an important concept that stem cells move towards the injury site in response to the signals coming from the injured cells (5, 6). This movement is in the direction of the signal gradient. They do not, however, affect areas or organs where such signals are absent. This has been confirmed by several research studies (7). The other fact that has clearly been elucidated and illuminated by the GFP positive cell studies is that adult stem cells have the ability to naturally transform into, or produce, cells of the skin, liver, lung, muscle, pancreas, heart and even the brain. (8)

This has disproved the long held dogma that adult stem cells have a limited capability to transform only into a select variety of cells, essentially just the ones they reside in, or at most, the cells of the developmental layer they arise from. (9) This is the dogma which dictated that hematopoietic stem cells can only produce cells of the blood lineage. Fortunately, recent research has put an end to this discussion. It has opened minds to explore further and opened doors to new possibilities.

In 2001, Dr. Diane S. Krause beautifully showed that even one adult bone marrow stem cell can completely reconstitute an entire blood system of red blood cells, lymphocytes and platelets with the help of the following ingenious experiments. (10)

Dr. Kraus and her team took 3 sets of female mice. They were all irradiated in order to kill their blood forming cells. Once cleared of their native blood and stem cells, the scientists injected the first set of mice with the marrow of a healthy, male mouse. Given the natural tendency of the hematologic stem cells to find their home in the marrow, they lodged and nestled in the marrow of the irradiated mouse. From there Dr. Krause was able to extract these isolated hematologic stem cells.

In the next step they injected only a single hematologic stem cell into each of the second set of irradiate female mice that were also free of native blood or stem cells. The third group of irradiated mice received neither marrow nor isolated stem cells. The results showed that all mice in the 3rd group that didn't receive any transplant died within 12 weeks, whereas the mice who received a single stem cell were able to re-constitute their entire blood composition (all different cell types) and lived a normal life span.

In addition, the team of scientists followed these surviving mice who received a single stem cell, for another few months. They searched for the Y-chromosome positive cells that could only have descended from that single male stem cell used to reconstitute the blood. To their surprise they found Y-chromosome positive cells in a variety of organs and tissues. These male cells found in the female mice clearly came from the single male stem cell transplant. This discovery was a major turning point in the perceptions of the plasticity and potential of the adult stem cells and served as the death nail in the long held belief that hematopoietic stem cells make only blood cells. In these experiments, a significant number of Y-chromosome positive cells were discovered in a large variety of tissues including, but not limited to stomach, colon, lung, skin, liver etc. (11)

These experiments proved that even one adult stem cell has the enormous capability to generate a large number of cells. They also confirmed that adult stem cell properties make them capable of leaving the marrow, sensing their way to a variety of tissues and organs, and then differentiating into cells of the local tissue. (12)

Since we cannot inject humans with glowing florescent stem cells like we do in mice, scientists had to come up with other ideas to confirm the above animal findings in humans. Serendipitously the gender-mismatched transplants (donor and recipient of different sexes) had already occurred in humans over the years. In the case of male patients receiving female organ transplant (liver, heart, lung), the recipient had the bone marrow repair system intact with all of its stem cells carrying XY (male) chromosomes whereas the donor organ had XX (female) chromosomes. Tissue biopsies and autopsies on these patients allowed the researchers to look for Y-chromosome positive cells in the donor organ. Finding the Y-positive cells in the female liver was proof that the male stem cells migrated to the donor organ and converted into cells of that tissue. In all patients who were tested, their liver contained 16%-43% Y-chromosome positive cells. (13, 14)

Similar findings were noted in female patients who received bone marrow transplants from male donors. Again in this case the organs of the female recipient had XX cells and the bone marrow transplant from a male had stem cells with XY chromosomes. When researchers looked for Y chromosome positive cells in the samples of their livers, they again found 5%-10% liver cells to be Y-chromosome positive, confirming their origin to be the donor bone marrow. (15) Many other gender-mismatched Y chromosome tracking studies revealed similar findings. Evidence of differentiated Y chromosome positive cells in the kidney, (16) lung, (17) heart, (18) and even the brain (19) was identified.

There is one more fascinating experiment that I want to tell you about which you are likely to find very interesting. It will also help you understand how stem cells work in general, even though we don't yet know the complete details of these processes.

In 2004, a simple, yet brilliant experiment was performed by Jang et al (20) to show how adult stem cells transform into differentiated cells. They took hematopoietic stem cells and some injured liver cells, placed them in a culture and separated the two with a semi-permeable membrane with pores large enough to allow the transfer of molecules, but too small for any cell movement across the membrane.

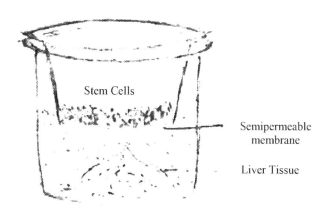

**Differentiation of Stem Cells into tissue cells**
**Experiment by Jang et al**

(Fig 6)

Within 8 hours, the Hematopoietic Stem Cells (HSCs) started transforming into liver cells and their number continued to increase with the passage of time. The experiment confirmed that micro environmental cues are responsible for conversion *in vitro*. The researchers also noted that the conversion to hepatic cells was minimal when undamaged liver cells were used and no change at all was noted when cells were cultured in the absence of liver tissue. This proved that there are molecular signals arising from the damaged liver cells which induce the adult stem cells to transform into the type of cells that are damaged. This feature of stem cells is not limited to liver cells alone. Stem cells respond in a similar fashion to signals from different types of damaged tissues in the body. Similarly, when HSCs were transplanted into liver-injured mice they converted into viable hepatocytes and the liver function was restored 2–7 days after transplantation. The Hematopoietic Stem Cells (HSCs) were responsible for regeneration of the injured liver by converting them into functional hepatocytes without fusion.

To recap what we have just learned:

- Adult stem cells can generate a large number and variety of cells.
- They respond to distant signals from damaged tissues in the body which mobilizes them from bone marrow and into the blood stream.

- Once near the damaged tissue they respond to molecular signals coming from damaged local cells.
- Based on the nature of these signals the stem cells transform into the cells that are damaged and need replacement.

Now let us bring in a few missing links and our story; "healing is an inside job" will be complete. The largest pool of stem cells in the body resides in the bone marrow. There is approximately one hematopoietic stem cell (HSC) for every 10,000 cells in bone marrow whereas blood only contains an average of 2,500 stem cells per ml., a significant dilution compared to the marrow. Recall that the marrow doesn't only contain Hematopoietic StemCells (HSCs) but also a variety of other pluripotent stem cells, (21) such as Mesenchymal Stem Cells (MSC). All of these cells have special receptors called CXCR4 that have high affinity for an agent called SDF-1; abundantly present in the marrow environment.

This affinity between CXCR4 and SDF-1 keeps the stem cells happily embedded in the marrow environment. In order to release and mobilize these stem cells the attraction between CXCR4 and SDF-1 must be overcome. This is accomplished by beckoning agents released from damaged tissues which reach the marrow via blood circulation. In the marrow these chemicals neutralize the marrow SDF-1, thus releasing the stem cells from their bond, freeing them to move and enter the blood stream. There are several agents that serve as the beckoning signal for the stem cells.

Two of the most common examples of these agents are Interleukin 8 (IL8) and Granulocyte Colony Stimulating Factor (GCSF), both are naturally present in the body and both can be commercially manufactured by pharmaceutical companies. (22,23) They are sometimes used in clinical practice to mobilize stem cells from the marrow. (More on this in the marrow transplant chapter). When these and similar molecules are released from the injured cells. They reach the marrow, break the bond between CXCR4 and SDF-1, and release the stem cells into the blood.

The stem cell journey starts here. The liberated stem cells jump into the blood. They dive into the rapid throws of a turbulent stream. Taking sharp turns, they reach the cyclone-like churning in the heart. Then, like a burst out of a dam they are pushed into the main outlet of the aorta. The stem cells are finally on their way to be delivered to the tissue in need. Moving rapidly through the arteries with their ever-reducing diameters, they navigate their way along a variety of blood cells, dodging parallel traffic, changing lanes and piloting sharp turns. This movement of stem cells from one part of the body to another area is called "trafficking".

When the stem cells are passing an injured area, they can sense the signals for assistance coming from the injured tissue. These signals are concentrated in the area of injury and include a type of SDF-1, (the same agent that the stem cell receptors (CXCR4) have high affinity for). By this time the stem cells are starting to crave their SDF partner and their CXCR4 receptors are hungry to latch on. When they find another SDF-1 at the injury site, they are highly attracted to it and move towards its highest concentration in a gradient-dependent fashion which directs the movement of stem cells towards the core of the injury. Once there, they quickly latch on to the local SDF-1 using their CXCR4 receptors, establishing a new home here, far from their old home in the marrow. To stem cells, home is where the SDF-1 is.

This process of localization to a new tissue at the injury site away from marrow is called "homing". SDF-1 is not the only factor involved in this homing process; many other molecules play a similar or complementary role. Once the stem cells are inside the damaged tissues, attracted by the SDF-1 gradient, the next step for them is to initiate their healing function.

As noted in the damaged liver experiment by Jang et al, a number of molecules and possibly cell-to-cell signaling mediates this step. The mechanism through which the stem cells accomplish this amazing task is not well understood but several known and possibly many more yet undiscovered agents are at work in this complex dance of repair and regeneration. What we do know and understand indicates that these stem cells start secreting growth factors and other molecules which stimulate the native pool of tissue stem cells. The latter, in turn, start multiplying and differentiating into damaged or lost cells. The newly arrived medics also seem to provide physical support and are often seen fused with the damaged cells. The exact stimulus for, or purpose of this fusion, is not yet clear to researchers. In addition, these stem cells themselves divide, both asymmetrically replenishing the stem cell pool, as well as differentiating into lost and damaged cells of the injured tissue. All these steps are still under investigation and may not be the only way stem cells accomplish their reparative and regenerative activity.

Let me confess that I have simplified the above steps about a thousand times. Many micro molecules and a number of complex steps are involved in the release, trafficking, homing, activation, secretion and trans-differentiation of the stem cells. However, unless you are planning a master's degree in stem cell science, these are not really important for you to learn. Research in this area is ongoing and extensive. The answers to complex questions are being routinely discovered. Once enough questions have been answered and put together like a million piece puzzle, a better and bigger picture of the mechanisms is likely to come into view. This hopefully will improve our understanding of how, when beckoned by silent signals from the injury site, do they sense, supply and service the need of the damaged tissue and how do stem cells respond, react, repair and resolve an injury.

It is also important to realize that SDF-1 is not only secreted by damaged tissue (where the concentration of SDF-1 is much higher) but it is also constantly released by major organs and tissues like the heart, brain, kidney, and liver. This promotes a continuous tissue renewal by stem cells. Higher concentrations of SDF-1 in the blood are noted after a heart attack (24), stroke (25), liver injury (26) and hypoxia.

A lack of oxygen supply to any tissue seems to be the trigger for the release of SDF-1 and therefore stem cell attraction. Understanding the SDF-1 and stem cell relationship explains why a higher number of stem cells in the blood, allows further stem cell movement along the SDF-1 gradient which translates into added regeneration and repair potential for the body.(27)

Several research studies have demonstrated that the number of circulating stem cells is an important indicator of recovery and regeneration. (28) A study by Tomoda et al reported that the higher the number of circulating stem cells at the time of a heart attack, the greater the recovery when compared to patients with lower baseline numbers of circulating stem cells. (29, 30) Similar results have been shown in stroke patients. (31)

Even though every step of this complex process is neither yet understood nor factually proven, one fact is for sure. Stem cells work and they work everytime. The evolving fields of regenerative medicine, stem cell science, genetics and tissue engineering hold the promise to expose, explain and exploit these processes for the benefit of humans and animals alike.

We are gaining more and more proof everyday that the use of adult stem cells from a patient's own body or cells from umbilical cord blood are safe and effective in several clinical conditions. Limitations persist and further investigations and ongoing oversight is required, but for those who argue that we don't know everything about adult stem cells so we ought not to use them at all, should read the history of medicine and its triumphs. Stem cells follow the same story line.

Centuries before the opioid receptors were discovered in the brain, gut or anywhere else, opium's ability to suppress pain was recognized and utilized, and it was no less effective than it is today. Later we claimed to have learned everything about opioids and produced pharmaceutical tablets and injections, only to be surprised by new discoveries of opoid receptors and mechanisms of action year after year. Similarly, senna and rhubarb, have worked for hundreds of years just the same as they do today. The only difference is, our ancestors knew they work and they work every time without any knowledge of receptors or nerves they stimulate to cause gut motility. They didn't even know there are nerves in the gut. Observation was the discoverer and experience was the teacher dictating safety and efficacy.

Edward Jenner or his contemporaries had no idea or understanding of an immune system or how cellular immunity works, but luckily, that didn't stop him from saving thousands of lives by vaccination in his own time and millions more since then. Similarly would you have stopped the use of penicillin because we didn't understand that penicillin inactivates the enzyme transpeptidase, necessary for cross-linking in the bacterial walls, which in turn disrupts the bacterial wall and kills it? Or that we didn't know if penicillin kills cocci or bacilli, gram negative or gram positive or aerobic or anaerobic organisms. What we did know and learn was that it can cure many infections in the skin, lung, urogenital tract and the brain. And as for the risk and benefits even after "everything" we now know about penicillin, still today, people around the world can die from penicillin use.

> *It is often necessary to make a decision on the basis of knowledge*
> *sufficient for action but insufficient to satisfy the intellect.*
> *~ Immanuel Kant*

# Chapter 13

# BONE MARROW TRANSPLANTS

*"How wonderful it is that nobody need wait a single moment before starting to improve the world." - Anne Frank*

Armed with the knowledge from animal experiments, that the bone marrow contains cells which can rebuild damaged or destroyed blood cells, a brave innovative physician took the next logical step. In 1956, Dr. Donnall Thomas used the infusion of bone marrow from a healthy twin into his sibling who was dying of leukemia and had undergone total body irradiation (bone marrow ablation to kill the cancer cells). (1) This treatment provided complete remission of the disease. Lack of billion dollar double blind studies, patented technology or FDA restrictions did not prevent the procedure and there were no religious activists blocking the hospital entrance citing interference in the "will of God".

This intuitive treatment, based on solid science, reason and rationale was not blocked, and a new chapter in medicine was written that changed the face of modern medicine. There is no doubt that since then multiple setbacks, failures, challenges and discoveries have helped improve the technique and enhanced our learning and understanding. Though not discovered or understood completely for some time, the treatment continued to work for these patients. New challenges continued to allow improvement and refinement of this life-saving procedure. Today Bone marrow transplantation is the most commonly practiced stem cell procedure in the world saving thousands of lives every day.

In 1958, a French scientist, Jean Dausset, discovered human histocompatibility antigens found on the surface of most cells in the body. (2) They serve as the identity card for own vs. foreign cells. This introduced the concept of histocompatibility or HLA matching between the transplant donor and recipient. A decade later in 1968, a successful bone marrow transplant between siblings was performed who had less than the identical matching of a twin.

In 1973, the first unrelated bone marrow transplant was reported to be successful, and that led to the first database of HLA-typed volunteer donors. A national donor registry finally became a reality in 1984 when congress passed the national organ transplant act. (3) Today you can search a registry of over 6 million volunteers for marrow or blood donors in 35 countries. But would any of this have happened if we were still doing mice and rabbit trials and waiting for pharmaceutical companies, till they found a way to patent the technology by undertaking billion dollar, decade long trials before some poor kid could take advantage of this treatment?

In 1990, Dr. Donnall Thomas won the Nobel Prize in medicine for his first human bone marrow transplant 34 years earlier, without FDA intervention, or legal and financial limitations of patent rights.

Today we understand that bone marrow transplant works because of its stem cell content not only of hematopoietic stem cells (HSC) but a variety of other stem cells. These cells have amazing plasticity and capability to repair and regenerate tissues all over the body. Methods are now available to measure and identify stem cells with the help of markers such as the cluster of differentiation (CD) on the surface of the cells. These stem cells can be taken from a patient, isolated, concentrated and either injected back into the patient, or they can be grown in a lab to increase their number. They can even be stored for later use, this often happens in current practice before a patient is irradiated for leukemia. The HSCs are removed from the patient's blood, and saved to be used after the irradiation to help rebuild the irradiated marrow; there is no risk of rejection, since the cells are the patient's own.

*The beginning of knowledge is the discovery of something*
*we do not understand. ~ Frank Herbert*

After 50 years, we still don't completely understand every step of this amazing recovery process but we know it works. It works not just in reconstituting the blood system but also lends a hand in the repair and regeneration of the other injured or diseased body tissues. The point to note is that despite the lack of complete understanding of the nature or mechanism of this recovery, bone marrow transplants have saved thousands of lives in the last half a century and continue to do so. The arguments against their use are gradually weakning, laws such as "Right to Try Act" which authorizes access to investigational drugs, biological products, and other treatments for terminal conditions are being passed in many states and countries providing legal protection to some procedures in a select group of patinets.

Not only have the bone marrow transplants served as a treatment option for patients who had no other option, they have also served as a source of study and experimentation in the stem cell field. A lot that we know about stem cells today was learned in practice from their use in bone marrow transplantation. Besides learning about stem cells and their potential to reconstitute the blood of an irradiated patient, we also learnt a lot about the constitution of the bone marrow transplant itself from studying these patients, their response and the nature and extent of stem cell incorporation in their body.

There is one other interesting and important fact about bone marrow transplant that we ought to explore here. When a patient receives any type of transplant, no matter how well matched, it is never a perfect match (unless from a twin). The cells of the transplanted organ are foreign to the patient's body and therefore, the body attacks them. This is a normal protective function of our immune system against foreign invader. In the transplantation scenario, however, it is not helpful for the body to attack the transplanted organ, leading to gradual destruction of the transplanted tissue. This is called "Host-vs-Graft Disease". Essentially, the immune system, in the bone marrow of the recipient (host) attacks the transplanted organ (graft). This leads to rejection of the organ; a common complication of all transplants. In order to prevent this rejection, transplant patients have to take immune suppressive drugs. These drugs do slow down the graft rejection, but they also leave the patient unprotected from other foreign invaders like bacteria, viruses, etc., which the immune system normally protects us from.

A different type of reaction scenario takes place in cases where the patient receives a marrow transplant rather than an organ transplant. Since the immune cells are a part of the marrow, when it is transplanted in a new host the immune cells in the marrow recognize the entire recipient as foreign and mount an immunologic attack. This is called "Graft-vs-Host Disease" (GvHD). (4) GvHD can cause blistering of the skin, intestinal hemorrhage and liver failure. Severe GvHD is extremely painful and fatal in up to 80 percent of the cases. It is the leading cause of transplant related mortality. Immunosuppressant drugs and steroids are often used to treat this serious complication. More recently, stem cell studies have discovered a beneficial role of Mesenchymal Stem Cells (MSC) in preventing or reducing the severity of GvHD. MSC have a recognized immune modulation effect and this property of mesenchymal stem cells has been exploited in the first stem cell based product approved in Canada. Prochymal® is the world's first approved drug which has stem cells as its active ingredient. Developed by Osiris Therapeutics Inc., it is indicated for the treatment of acute graft-vs-host disease (GvHD). According to the product's literature "Prochymal is truly an off-the-shelf stem cell product that is stored at the point-of-care and infused through a simple intravenous line without the need to type match or immunosuppress the recipient".

Established scientific proof is now on the table, that MSCs, even from an Allogeneic source (as in Prochymal®) are not immunogenic. (5) They do not induce the rejection reaction; they actually prevent it. Years of research and practice has also established that autologous MSC from the patient are safe and provide some level of benefit in many ailments. (6) Information about the exact nature and extent in specific diseases will only come from experience. Safe, frequent and unrestricted use of the autologous stem cells for treatment, involving observation and collection of data in human subjects will certainly help progress the field in a practical and meaningful way from animal testing to real cures.

> *"The real voyage of discovery consists not in seeking*
> *new landscapes, but in having new eyes." ~ Marcel Proust*

I am definitely not proposing that medical treatments or procedures should not be regulated, quite the opposite. I believe that toxic synthetic substances that are completely unnatural and alien to human bodies (most of the current pharmaceuticals) should be highly regulated. Treatments that hardly cure anything or alleviate suffering, just delay the inevitable by a few days or weeks, devoid of any quality of life.... Yes! They should be strictly regulated and their usefulness measured against their physical and fiscal cost. There should be strict oversight and requirement for open disclosure of such "advance treatments" that wreak havoc on the bodies already weakened by the disease and make the final days miserable with no possibility of cure, remission or even relief. They claim exuberant costs from the family and take an enormous physical toll on the patient, so of course they should be regulated.

However, when it comes to natural, proven, safe and beneficial, though not completely understood treatments, there ought to be different criteria and approaches. Using one's own cells for treatment is not the same as ingesting a highly toxic chemical substance for treatment. When enough scientific knowledge has been amassed, and safety has been confirmed by use, the practice should be allowed to develop and take its natural course. With good, scientific knowledge, and research experience, a safe treatment plan can be carried out with minimal risks though potential benefits. Freedom from restrictive control should be granted in such cases so that the science doesn't go underground and patients are not forced to travel abroad and fall into the hands of completely unregulated, unscrupulous and opportunistic providers and practices. This is especially true when it comes to diseases that have no cure. When the burden of suffering is too heavy, compassionate use of relatively safe treatments that are well-supported by clinical evidence should be liberal, but of course after a well-informed consent process.

However, the same cannot be said about the use of stem cells from other external sources. For example, an allogeneic transplant from another person can involve rejection or transmission of infection and disease as significant risks. Additionally, any significant manipulation of these cells outside the body may carry the risk of contamination and structural changes in their DNA that may have serious consequences, such as introduction of a viral infection or the development of cancer. Further studies and trials are needed. We will discuss this in more detail in the specific disease treatment chapters.

The same is true for cells that are not naturally present in the body, such as embryonic stem cells (ESC) that have known tumorigenic properties.

There is no documented evidence of safety and not enough data to support their efficacy. Ongoing research on ESC to explore and understand the ways they develop into differentiated cells and studies to establish safety are very important. They may be a valuable ore in a gold mine of knowledge but not safe to use in their raw form.

Even more important are such insights for iPS cells that are completely unnatural since they are externally manipulated into doing something that cells are naturally programmed not to do (go back in evolution towards embryonic state). This is not to understate the potential these cells hold. In fact, iPS cells may possibly hold the most potential for future use in medicine.... not necessarily for injection into the body but to study the development of diseases, the discovery of drugs and treatment as well as the production of healing factors.

AUTOLOGOUS TISSUE TRANSPLANTATION:

*"Imagination is more important than knowledge.*
*Knowledge is limited. Imagination encircles the world."*
*~Albert Einstein*

Autologous tissues have been used in medical and surgical treatments in humans for centuries. Reports of healthy skin and fat grafts to battle wounds and injuries are noted in Greek medicine. A fat and skin transfer for reconstructive use or burn care is itself a century old practice. Use of cadaver bone and ligament used in orthopaedic surgeries and reconstruction procedures also has a long history, and we have even longer experience with blood transfusions from both autologous and allogeneic donors.

Not only the marrow, but other tissues such as the leg veins in heart bypass surgeries, bone graft in spine surgeries, autologous blood transfusion for blood loss during surgery, skin grafting for burns and fat grafting for wound healing or reconstructive surgery, are all autologous tissue transplant techniques safely practiced in medicine today and for more than half a century with documented benefits. The use of hematopoietic stem cells from marrow or mesenchymal stem cells from fat is no different and should have no additional restrictions if taken from and used on the same patient (autologous). (7, 8)

Numerous studies and case reports from around the world have documented the successful use of umbilical cord-derived allogeneic mesenchymal stem cells, without any report of rejection. The significant immune, privilege nature of these cells has been confirmed by many clinical studies and clinical trials have confirmed the safety of these adult stem cells in clinical use. (9, 10)

I don't buy into conspiracy theories or unwarranted paranoia of every for-profit venture. There is nothing wrong in making money, within reason, on a good product. But when it comes to how our healthcare system and research structure is designed to restrict and limit physicians; the only professionals educated, trained and experienced to render treatments, it makes me wonder why people who are not qualified, trained or experienced in patient care, are directing what the physicians can and cannot do.

To understand any action, you need to understand the underlying motive. The scientific research field in the USA is a multi-billion dollar a year industry. Many researchers spend more time writing grants and working on how and where to get more money to have their own labs, rather than doing true scientific work. Like I said earlier, there is no apple grove without a few bad apples. Every year they demand even bigger budgets, while sometimes promoting meaningless research that earns them a spot on the evening news and larger bundles of public and private funding, but little in the way of useable science.

It is like convincing the common man that measuring water by a cup, or liter, or gallon, or cc is not a scientific way to measure. We must report it as the number of molecules of $H_2O$ to be scientific because in patient care, accuracy matters. Whether this has any practical significance or not has become a point of debate. If this idea is adopted, it will give these labs a huge project paying them millions in return and eventually a patented method to report how much water by number of molecules every patient drinks. You and I will pay the cost of it with no benefit what-so-ever.

By opposing every simple way to reach clinical use, they make the road to clinics run through their labs, rewarding them with millions in the process. The system has become so convoluted that bringing any ideas to a patient takes a long, tortuous, and extremely expensive route. The real scientists and researchers who are making discoveries and breaking new ground are often funded by the pharmaceutical and biotechnology companies. These companies are patenting those discoveries, adding to their bottom line. This, however, makes the final treatment more and more expensive. If something is not patentable, no one has an interest in it, but there is still fierce objection to its use because it will take away the market share of these companies.

I am a believer of the Occam's razor philosophy of parsimony and succinctness, a preference in a simple, scientific method as it is historically explained. (11) It is a good principle to explain any phenomenon by the simplest hypotheses possible. More contemporary explanation acknowledges that the simplest answer is not always correct but the researchers should avoid stacking up theories to prove a hypothesis if a simple explanation fits the observation. Today, scientists are not interested in simple answers. They are interested in patentable answers. No matter how complex or expensive it makes a simple act.

Let us say for example, in the following metaphor, using vitamin C will not be acceptable, as it doesn't have the same number of scientific studies that a patented new "vitamin-C-like" molecule has, which has been tested in 2000 patients spending millions of dollars and shows 20 % better results than a placebo. Well, that is pretty pathetic because what it means is that 80% of the people get no benefit, but it is a statistically significant difference so the FDA will grant it approval. The natural vitamin C which is not patentable but effective in most patients will no longer be used and labeled as "unscientific".

This is how they debunk all simple, natural and common-sense solutions as non-scientific because no one spent millions of dollars to publish dozens of papers in its support. Though doctors have good clinical experience with it and patients have benefited time after time, these simple and natural treatments are blocked in favor of completely unnatural, synthetic, chemical molecules that have to be tested for both efficacy and safety and must rightfully have years of studies to make sure they are safe for human consumption. But of course they are patentable.

Even if a safe and natural alternative is present, doctors are not permitted to use it. They are forced to prescribe this new "standard of care" chemical because it has the FDA seal of approval. This sad state of affairs was eerily predicted by

President Dwight Eisenhower in his final address to the nation. He expressed his concern for corruption of the scientific process as part of the centralization of funding in the Federal government. (12)

> "The prospect of domination of the nation's scholars by Federal employment, project allocations, and the power of money, is ever present – and is gravely to be regarded. Yet, in holding scientific research and discovery in respect, as we should, we must also be alert to the equal and opposite danger that public policy could itself become the captive of scientific-technological elite"………President Dwight Eisenhower, Final Address, January 17, 1961.

I believe we have reached that time already. Independent universities have increasingly become controlled by providers of financial grants. This is stifling, free, scientific thought. Research has become a complex and costly endeavor focused more on coming up with a unique way that can be patented and commercialized rather than a useful way that will provide a simple and practical solution. Pharmaceutical industry and their highly paid research scientists are not interested in any cure that may close their pipeline of drugs which maintains patients in a diseased state, managing their symptoms thus growing the number of users for their products. Imagine if a stem cell cure for diabetes is discovered and insulin producing beta cells could be injected into the pancreas of patients with diabetes; no one will buy the billions of diabetes pills a month…. billions of injections of insulin, glucometers, supplies and all the billions of dollars worth of products used to treat the complications of diabetes, kidney failure requiring dialysis and its associated products, machines, chemicals, drugs, etc…etc..etc.. Hope you get the picture and the motivation behind the actions I mentioned earlier.

# Chapter 14

# REGENERATIVE MEDICINE

**Prometheus and the Salamander**

On the outskirts of Mexico City, in a lake, resides one of the most unusual species; the Axolotl Salamander that spends its entire life in a larval form, never maturing, thus capable of regenerating any of its body parts. Axolotl is not alone in this ability. Most members of the salamander family have this regenerative capability. In fact, limb and organ regeneration is common among organisms, both in the plant and animal kingdom. Crayfish, earthworms, frogs, starfish and planarian are a few common examples. (1)

Observation of this regenerative capability is also not new; ancient people had observed, documented and developed myths about this unusual capacity of certain organisms and organs. According to Greek mythology, Prometheus suffered the wrath of Zeus for steeling fire from the Gods and giving it to humans. As a punishment, he was tied to a boulder and an eagle feasted on his liver all day; during the night the liver regenerated so that the eagle could eat it again. It is interesting that of all the vital organs, this myth involves the liver. As we now know, human liver has the highest regenerative capacity of any organs. In fact it seems to be the only human organ that can regrow to a normal size only from a fraction of its tissue. This has been taken as an indication that the Greeks knew about the regenerative ability of liver that differentiates it from other vital organs. Whether this assumption is true or not, the ancient myths do incorporate the concept of regeneration of all or part of an organism from its remnants.

Hydra is another example from Greek mythology; a character that Hercules had to kill as the second of his twelve labors. According to the story, this monster of the sea had multiple heads and if one head was cut off it regrew new heads in its place. Now there exists a primitive animal species that has been named after this mythological character, because it possesses, in real life, the same ability to regrow new heads and it can develop into a many-headed organism much like the mythological hydra. If its body is cut in half, the lower half will grow a new head, and the upper half will grow a new foot. If the head and foot are both cut off, a new head and foot will grow, and the Hydra will maintain its original polarity. Because of this unique ability, Hydra is one of the most commonly studied regenerating organisms. (1)

It appears that the less complex organisms have more, remarkable, regenerative ability. One such example is Planarian; it is a family of flatworms which have been studied for their remarkable, regenerative capacity. (2) If a Planarian worm is cut into two, each half regrows to form a complete Planarian. Even if the worm is cut into hundred pieces, each piece can form a whole new worm genetically identical to the original. It appears that in hydra, planarian and even in salamander, there are special kinds of cells that are primitive or developmental in origin and that have the ability to either revert to their embryonic code or are able to maintain their early developmental coding throughout the life of the organism. (3)

What happened to our regenerative abilities? Fact is, we also possess regenerative capabilities, just not to the extent of a planarian or a salamander. Think of all the times you fell off a bicycle scraping your knees, cut yourself with a kitchen knife or may be broke a bone playing sports. How do you think the wounds healed? It is the regenerative capacity of those tissues that help you mend your body. If you lose a finger nail it will grow back. Even if you chop off a little bit of the tip of a finger it will likely grow back as long as there is not too much loss of tissue. Besides the skin and bones, the liver and blood also have significant regenerative ability. Especially important is the body's ability to constantly produce new red and white blood cells, both of which wear out and die, so a new supply is constantly needed to nourish and protect the body.

Why do some tissues regenerate better than others? How do they regenerate at all? And can we improve this regenerative capacity of the human body? All these make interesting questions that do not yet have clear answers. Stem cell research and medical trials are leading us to answers and solutions that may one day allow us to grow limbs and organs or at least repair the ones that get damaged.

## New Lease on Life

When I was, may be 8 years old, my uncle brought us a train from Scotland. It was one of those fancy toys with an elaborate setup of railroads, stations, fire hydrants, bridges, the whole nine yards. It was our favorite toy and our most prized possession. My brothers and I played and over-played with it until one day the train didn't start. It took jerks but didn't move, even though the rest of the accessories, the cart it pulled and the bridges it passed, were all in good condition.

We changed the battery, we cleaned it, and poked around in its mechanical belly, but nothing… my younger brother said "our train died". For days the whole setup sat in one corner of the living room, being mourned. We occasionally moved the train manually from here to there as if attending its wake but not yet ready to declare the funeral.

Then an astonishing thing happened, one of my Dad's friends was visiting us, and saw the train sitting in the corner. He tried to turn it on, which of course it did not. He then flipped it over, took out his key chain attached to a small knife, and opened the cover. I was watching him from a distance hoping he wouldn't break our broken train. He worked on the engine for a few minutes, closed the cover, put it back on the track and turned it on. To my amazement, it blew its familiar whistle and started moving. I was the first to run and pick it up, turned it off and turned it on again. It worked just like before. I asked my Dad's friend, "What did you do?" He said, "I gave it a new lease on life". Those words rang in my head for some time. I did not know the meaning of lease then, but "new lease on life" had a nice ring to it and to my ears it was whistling music.

The next time, when I was asked to write an essay about my future aspirations, I wrote "I want to be a doctor, so I can give my patients a new lease on life". Unfortunately when I did become a doctor, I realized it is not nearly as easy as fixing a train. In fact, most times we barely can extend that lease, much less renew it. Regenerative medicine has the potential to make that dream come true. Replace or regenerate a dying organ and give the entire body a new life.

## Paradigm Shift in Modern Medicine

Today the best hope we have for serious illnesses involves replacing a failing organ like a heart or kidney or liver with a borrowed organ from a donor. The problem is the huge shortage of donated organs, for every 20-25 patients needing an organ only one actually gets it and even that is not an ideal match. So the patient has to take immune suppressant drugs for the rest of his life. Despite that, the organ is slowly rejected anyway, and the patient is back to square one. On top of that, there are many organs that cannot be replaced, like the brain or spinal cord. We do have a work around for this problem though; instead of replacing the entire organ we can only replace the part or the cells that are diseased or damaged.

A century ago, transplanting a heart from one person to another was a subject of science fiction. A decade ago, fashioning a new bladder or a new trachea (wind pipe) out of a patient's own cells was just as unrealistic. Today they are all realities. What a difference a few years can make in technological advancement. Within the last decade, advances in the ability to grow, and redirect stem cells into a variety of specific cell lines has completely changed the playing field.

New knowledge of a rich supply of regenerative cells in our bodies has changed the focus from external sources of stem cells to our own stem cells. Additionally, better understanding of the plasticity and safety profile of adult stem cells (ASCs) has led to a rapid increase in the number of adult stem cell clinical trials. Most common type of ASC is Hematopoietic Stem Cells (HSC) from the bone marrow. Another abundant type of ASCs, known as Mesenchymal stem cells (MSCs), are present in many tissues though are easiest to extract from the bone marrow and adipose tissue (fat). Several biotechnology companies are now working on using MSCs and HSCs for developing new treatments for a range of diseases.

ASCs, fortunately, don't have the ethical or legal baggage that some of the other stem cells do. Their safety has also been established for several decades both in allogeneic and autologous use during bone marrow transplants. ASCs, especially MSCs, have been shown to have the capacity to differentiate into a variety of specialized cell types including heart, liver, cartilage, bone, and muscle cells.

Like most other stem cells they have also been shown to secrete growth promoting, immune modulating, and anti-inflammatory substances that assist in the healing and the regenerative process. Regenerative medicine advances are making use of all the different functions of stem cells. Besides cellular therapy, where cells themselves are used as treatment, other regenerative medicine technologies involve tissue engineering and genetically-engineered stem cell transplantation.

**Regenerative Medicine: What can we expect?**

- A burn or wound gets a spray of stem cells and heals in less than a week without scars.
- A stem cell injection in AIDS patients kills the HIV and prevents further infection.
- A heart attack patient gets an injection of factors that reprogram cardiac scar tissue into beating heart cells—avoiding complications.
- A patient with Alzheimer's disease takes a pill of stem cell growth factors that instructs the patient's brain to repair or replace injured neurons.
- A bladder or urethra destroyed in an accident is grown in a lab and surgically placed in the patient without risk of rejection.
- A lung destroyed by cancer is grown in a bioreactor using the patient's own cells and then transplanted in their chest.

The sky is the limit; human curiosity and our brain's innovative potential may lead us to treatments and solutions that you and I cannot even imagine today.

> *Curiosity is lying in wait for every secret.*
> *- Ralph Waldo Emerson*

Regenerative medicine is an exciting branch of scientific and clinical research and practice which deals with engineering, replacement and/or regeneration of human cells, tissues or organs, to restore normal functions. It refers to a group of biomedical approaches to clinical therapies that usually involve the use of stem cells. The field may be new but its scope expands from a simple injection of a patient's own cells to complete human organs grown in a lab. It is the new frontier of medicine that has the potential to benefit millions of people. (4)

# Chapter 15

# TISSUE ENGINEERING

**Tissue:** An aggregate of cells forming a definite kind of structure with a specific function.

**Engineering:** The action of working artfully to bring something about.

**Tissue engineering:** Artfully fashioning a combination of cells, and other materials, with suitable biochemical factors to improve or replace biological functions.

This may mean using cells to:

1 - Replace damaged or diseased functional cells.
2 - Develop new biologic tissues to replace damaged or lost tissues or organs, or
3 - Build in part or whole of an organ in a lab to be transplanted in a body.

*Everything in the universe is within you. Ask all from yourself.*
*~ Rumi*

A number of individuals have been credited with the coinage of this term. However it appears that it may have been invented a few times independently before it became broadly accepted and adopted. Regardless of who coined it, its meaning has evolved with time, as technology took exhilarating wild turns over the years; it has opened doors to possibilities that were sci-fi at best, only a few years ago.

Until 1858, Schleiden and Schwann's theory of spontaneous cell generation from spontaneous formation of crystals was the prevailing belief. (1) Virchow refuted this old concept and described cell formation with the famous words, "omniscellula e cellula..." cells arise from pre-existing cells. (2) This brought about the idea that tissue regeneration is dependent on cell proliferation, ensuing research focused at a more fundamental cellular level, resulting in the discovery of a variety of other tissues. From that point on, researchers experimented with growing cells outside the body.

This started with simple organisms like bacteria and moved on to larger animals, until lab growth of human cells became possible. However, it was not until 1998, with the development of human embryonic stem cell lines, that the basis of modern tissue engineering was formed. (3) The growth and progress in this area has been exponential. In 1984, there was only one published article with the term "tissue engineering" in it; in 2014 alone, there were more than 100,000 articles about tissue engineering.

A soft acrylic, human-like material has been successfully used for years in humans for lens implant in a cataract afflicted eye and is probably the earliest example of bio engineering,. In modern terms however, tissue engineering involves an inter-disciplinary approach with the goal of growing tissues or organs, directly from an individual's own cells. This approach envisions "human", not "human-like", tissues and promises to eliminate the common problem of donor tissue rejection.

Tissue engineering is still in its infancy. However, indications are strong that in the future it may be possible to engineer replacements for most tissues. Today engineered tissues in principle can replace any biological tissue damaged by disease or injury. Though not all applications have been adequately investigated or clinically tested, at least 25 or so procedures are currently using tissue-engineered systems in clinical practice.

Tissue engineering requires four basic ingredients:

1 - Cells: Can be derived from embryonic, induced pluripotent or adult stem cell sources.

2 - Supporting Matrix: Such as collagen and hyaluronic acids or alginate scaffolds. (4)

3 - Growth factors: Platelet-derived growth factor, fibroblast growth factor, transforming growth factor-β and epidermal growth factor are common examples. (5)

4 - Bioreactor: To maintain specific temperature, pH, mechanical stresses and biochemical gradients. (6)

Cells, as you know, are the building blocks of tissue, which form the organs and structure of a body. Groups of cells make and secrete their own support structures, called extra-cellular matrix. This matrix serves as a scaffold for them to grow on. The process of tissue engineering begins with building this scaffold from a variety of materials. Cells supplemented with growth factors are then introduced into the scaffold, which in the presence of the right environment develop into a tissue.

Newer methods are using a mixture of cells, scaffolds, and growth factors, incubated together, which allows them to "self-assemble." In the approach described below, an existing scaffold was used from a donor organ that was stripped off its cells, leaving a collagen scaffold that was used to grow a new trachea. This approach, using scaffolding from human tissue, holds great promise to make customized organs from a patient's own cells and supporting structures, which would not be rejected. This process has already been used to bioengineer the trachea, heart, liver, lung, and kidney tissues. (7)

New biomaterials are also constantly being developed. They are designed to direct and promote the growth, differentiation and organization of cells in order to form tissues. Earlier in their evolution, biomaterials were derived from animal sources, the earliest example is the sub mucosa, derived from porcine small intestine, which has been used as a scaffold material in over half a million patients.

Experimentally engineered tissues include artificial bladders, urethra, and trachea and so on. With the advent of nanotechnology, the engineering component is getting integrally involved in the whole process. Scientists are using a variety of innovative techniques to develop a number of useful tissues. Nano-engineers at the University of California, San Diego, have just disclosed a new biomaterial for repairing damaged human tissue, which doesn't wrinkle up when stretched; it, therefore, mimics the properties of native human tissue. (8) A research group at the University of Arkansas, in June of 2014, reported developing a biomaterial that can regenerate damaged skeletal muscle. Others have successfully used stem cells and pluripotent cells to make bone tissue in the lab, which is compatible with surgical use in patients. (9, 10)

Examples of such innovative feats are becoming common place; however, the most amazing products of tissue engineering remain the whole organs developed in a lab. One such recent occasion, when people around the globe held their cumulative breath in awe, was the day when Claudia Castillo, a mother of two young children, was saved by an engineered windpipe (trachea) built in a lab in Bristol, UK. In this amazing procedure Dr. Hollander and Professor Birchall's team used a trachea from a cadaver, removed its cells using chemicals to expose the supporting tissue scaffold, while the patient's own stem cells, removed from her bone marrow, were used to line and seed this scaffold. This three dimensional tube was then incubated in a bioreactor developed in Milan, Italy. In the next four days the cells penetrated the scaffold tissue and generated the linings of the trachea. The newly devised trachea was then flown to Barcelona, Spain, and transplanted into the patient by Professor Paolo Macchiarini.

This international collaboration succeeded in replacing Claudia's own trachea that was destroyed by tuberculosis and was slowly killing her. The results were nothing less than miraculous; the engineered trachea was incorporated in the tissues, blood vessels grew into it and it functioned perfectly, saving her life.

While surgeons are replicating this success in other hospitals, here at home Dr. Anthony Atala of the Regenerative Medicine Institute at Wake Forest University has been fashioning new 3D bladders out of the patients' own cells. These are incubated in a bioreactor and transplanted back successfully in the patients. The body does not even notice that a foreign object has been installed; this sleight of hand works, because the bladders, like Claudia's trachea, are lined with the patient's own cells, so they resemble the "self", escaping any immune attack. These bladders have been successfully working in patients for several years. Wake Forest Laboratory has continued to replicate this success, also made new urethras, and is reportedly working on a variety of other organ regenerations including kidney tissue.

The organs that have been developed in a lab and used in patients include blood vessels, ureters, bladders, skin grafts, cartilage, and trachea. More complex organ tissues like the heart, lung and liver have also been successfully created in the lab, but they are a long way from being easily reproduced or ready for use in a patient.

Although organ generation is a complex process, the tissue engineering methods described above, raise the hope to treat organ failure in humans in the future. Besides adult stem cells and embryonic stem cells, induced pluripotent stem cells hold the potential for cell replacement and organ generation. Labs around the world are tirelessly working on these and other techniques; the proof of concept has been demonstrated for a variety of tissue regenerations. Research in this field is burgeoning and is highly promising with progressive developments in technology, inching closer to clinics.

# Chapter 16

# CONCEPT TO CLINIC: Part I

The role of Stem Cells in Cardiovascular Diseases:

Our world, and especially the United States of America, is going through a major healthcare challenge. Like most western countries our population is aging. This growth in the number and proportion of older adults is unprecedented. Two factors—longer life spans and aging baby boomers—will combine to double the population of Americans aged 65 years or older during the next 25 years to about 72 million.

By 2030, older adults will account for roughly 20% of the U.S. population. (1) By 2050, it is anticipated that Americans aged 65 or older, will number nearly 89 million people, or more than double the number of older adults we had in the United States in 2010. (2) This increase in the aging population increases the burden of disease, which means more chronic diseases and degenerative illnesses. Along with the suffering comes the stress on the economy. Our nation's healthcare expenditures are already the highest among developed countries, and are steadily on the rise. Most of this cost is related to the management of chronic diseases. Health economists warn that the cost of healthcare for persons aged 65 or older is 3-5 times higher than for someone younger than 65. (3)

Take a look at the prevalence of some of the common diseases in the United States. You will realize that it is some miracle that a few of us are still walking around disease free. The numbers add up to be more than the entire USA population because some unfortunate ones among us have more than one disease or its complications. Let us have a look at our disease burden.

**29.1 million Diabetes.** (5)

1.3 million HIV infections. (14)

1,275,000 spinal cord injuries. (17)

500,000 have Crohn's disease

25,000 live with ALS

73 million in the US have high blood pressure.

36 million people suffer cardiovascular diseases.

53 million adults carry a diagnosis of arthritis.

5.2 million have Alzheimer's disease.(6)

1 million have Parkinson's disease.(7)

**5 million adults live with COPD.**(8)

**400,000 have Multiple Sclerosis.**

**795,000 suffer a stroke every year.**

**39.5 million suffer from Asthma.**(9)

1.7 million sustain a TBI annually.(11)

15 million have some type of cancer. (10)

20 million suffer from peripheral neuropathy.

5.5 million have connective tissue disease.(15)

7 million plus, have some kind of chronic liver disease.

20 million patients live with chronic kidney disease. (16)

**1.4 million suffer from Inflammatory Bowel Diseases.** (13)

**59 million have low back pain; 30.1 millionsuffer neck pain.**

Millions more are diagnosed with one of these ailments each year. Note that these are just the chronic illnesses without a cure which require ongoing care and management. The price tag for these reaches trillions of dollars a year. This does not take into account any of the infectious diseases like pneumonia, or meningitis, it is without considering migraines or muscle pains, without mentioning peptic ulcers or pancreatitis, prostate or bladder issues and not even including congenital deformities or nutritional deficiency diseases.

No wonder hospitals are always full and we spend 17% of the nation's GDP on healthcare. A bigger concern is that these diseases are not decreasing in incidence. The cost of care is escalating, our population is aging and more of us are living with these diseases. Medicare spending is projected to increase from $555 billion in 2011 to $903 billion in 2020. (4) It is clear that if we don't find a way to improve the health of this aging population and reduce the morbidity associated with the leading chronic diseases, the social and economic consequences will be disastrous. Improved diet, life style, exercise and preventive care all certainly help and should be encouraged but there also needs to be a drastic change in the way our healthcare system works. Ours is a model of disease, we diagnose and treat diseases, for most of which we only have symptomatic management, not cures.

So what is the solution? Our current healthcare practice model clearly isn't the solution. The way our healthcare is designed around diagnosis and management of disease, there is a disincentive for preventions and cures. In fact, there is a trillion dollar incentive to prevent cures from happening and keep managing diseases. Think about it. If today we find a cure for high blood pressure or diabetes, billions of dollars a month worth of medication and product sales will stop. Trillions of dollars worth of management cost for their complications will also stop.

If your business is selling medicines, what would you want? A one-time cure or a daily treatment, that runs year after year? What's more, it will also stop billions of dollars going to basic research labs for animal and chemical testing of these pharmaceutical treatments, which people forget is just as big of a business and it will shut down if we start finding cures for major health problems. It shouldn't then be a surprise to see the money being spent on lobbying and mounting resistance against the "stem cell cures". Unfortunately money does talk. The only way out of this quagmire is to educate the masses to demand the safe forms of these treatments and demand them soon. With the new discovery of the natural healing system of stem cells we need to develop a model of disease prevention based on the maintenance of optimal health rather than waiting for diseases to appear before an intervention is carried out.

We know how to measure the stem cell count, we know that a higher stem cell count translates into better health and we know several ways to increase and maintain the healthy stem cell count (see healthy stem cell lifestyle chapter). Additionally, advancing our understanding of stem cells in each organ, their role in regeneration, and their clinical applications to replace or enhance lost functions, is likely to give exponential results. Of course we are not there yet, but if supportive policies are adopted, rapid progress in this field is expected, that will usher in the promising days of better healthcare.

In practical terms, though human embryonic stem cells (hESC) technically have huge potential to become any cell in the body, the challenges to their use are just as huge. To begin with:

1 - The acquisition of hESC is a socially-charged, ethically-controversial, and financially-challenging endeavor.

2 - Secondly, by definition, hESC is a cell that when implanted in an animal is able to produce tumors called Teratoma which has tissues from all three embryonic germ layers. So basically hESC must have the potential to form tumors, which can be a risk when we don't know how it will act once introduced in the body.

3 - Thirdly, the hESC are always derived from embryos that don't have the same genetic makeup as the prospective patient so they are allogeneic, with the possible risk of rejection.

4 - Due to funding restrictions and ethical objections, the hESC research has not progressed as well or as far as Adult Stem Cell (ASC) research has, so we have limited experience with these cells and we are farther from their meaningful clinical use.

Induced Pluripotent Stem Cells (iPS cells) have now provided a possible stand in for the hESC and a new era of cell reprogramming technology is underway. This may very possibly overcome the challenges hESC have historically faced. However, this too is not free of difficulties. As discussed in the iPS cell chapter, the cost, time, cancer risk and the possibility of auto-reprogramming after introduction in a patient, remain a significant concern.

In every dark cloud there is a silver lining. When the restrictions on hESC research started suffocating scientific curiosity and blocking the quest for knowledge, scientists looked for alternatives and the research in Adult Stem Cells (ASC) blossomed. Innovative new approaches started evolving. This has given us more experience with the ASC than any other type of stem cell. More research studies and clinical trials are underway in the USA and around the globe using ASC rather than hESC, UCSC and iPS cells combined. ASC do carry several advantages.

1 - They are not controversial.
2 - Their cancer-forming potential is less than other pluripotent cells.
3 - They are autologous (from the patient) with no risk of rejection.
4 - They are cheaply and readily available from any patient.

Their challenges are, that they are few in numbers in any tissue and are difficult to find and identify. Their plasticity or ability to differentiate into a variety of cell types is suspected to be less than the hESC. In an emergency situation they are not quickly available in large numbers.

On the other hand we have extensive experience with these cells due to their half a century long use in bone marrow transplants. Therefore, all things considered, adult stem cells have the best chance of going from concept to clinic, faster than any other type of stem cell. Let's look at individual diseases, the challenges they pose and the possibilities stem cells provide in their treatment, management or cure.

## THE U-TURN

"What do you call the student who graduates last from the medical school graduating class?" asked my director. Having heard it a thousand times before and already perturbed with the long argument, I mumbled, "Doctor". "Then stop acting like you are better than the rest of them and get back to work," he scowled. That was the last argument I had with my program director at the University Hospital in New York, where I was an intern in the plastic surgery training program, itching to get out.

I graduated at the top of my medical school class and had excellent test scores. Following my painfully competitive nature I applied for one of the most sought-after specialty of plastic surgery at prestigious institutions across the USA. I was on cloud nine when I got accepted at the Staten Island University Hospital in New York. I packed my old faithful Toyota Celica with all my belongings, accompanied by my best friend; we drove from Dallas to the northeast. I dropped my buddy off in Worcester at Mass General Hospital for his cardiology training and jumped back in my car shouting, "New York, here I come."

Plastic surgery may be glamorous in the end but it also begins with the medical slavery, in general surgery called internship. First few days passed in excitement, and then the exhaustion, sleep deprivation and loads of menial labor started to take its toll.

Surgeons are a unique breed of practitioners. They are skilled, strong-willed, focused, dedicated, and industrious. Good bedside manners and compassionate conversations, however, are generally not their strong suit. We did our morning rounds around 6 a.m. marking body parts to be operated that day, taking notes on patients and procedures. By the time the patient was fully awake we were out of the door.

We would see that patient a few hours later in the operating room already under anesthesia. After verifying the patient's identity and checking the marks we made earlier we would grab the scalpel-- to be honest, the only thing I grabbed was the retractors for my seniors who did the actual surgeries. After spending hours in the operating room, standing silently, crushing one foot with the other to stay awake, the surgery would finally be over. The operating surgeon would leave the room for me to close the sutures; like the lions leave their kill after they had their fill, for the hyenas to feed off the remains.

After grabbing a quick bite it was time for more surgeries. This was followed by evening rounds which mostly entailed looking at wounds from the previous day surgeries, but in and out just as fast as the morning rounds. Some of it is not the surgeon's fault; our health care system has turned hospitals into assembly lines.

In any case, I used to get home, or to my basement in someone else's home, late at night. Eat a bowl of cereal and crash. This daily routine was broken only by every fourth night call which meant 32 continuous hours instead of the regular 12, easily making it a 100 hour week. What was even more difficult and discouraging was the fact that I didn't really know any of the patients. Our history-taking was brief and only focused on the surgical problem. The general medicine doctors did the detailed evaluation to clear the patient for surgery and anesthesiologists did their own assessment and medication history. One of the surgical residents would go in between tasks and get the patient or family to sign the surgical consent while I saw the patients waking up on morning rounds, waking up again on evening rounds and in between, sleeping on the operating table. I felt no bond with my patients.

I remember being disillusioned. Soon I realized that I didn't have a "surgeon's personality". I needed more human contact and interaction with patients. I wanted to treat my patients holistically, not only nail their fracture or remove their appendix. As valuable as these procedures are, clearly, my desire to be the kind of physician I wanted to be, was not going to be fulfilled there. I found myself questioning why I was there. Why was I trying to be a plastic surgeon? As the answer came to me so did the realization that I was there for the wrong reasons. I didn't want to be a plastic surgeon; I wanted to prove that I could be a plastic surgeon. I was trying to show that I had made it where most people dream to go. That competitiveness only hurt me. I finally learned that the only one I needed to compete with was I, to strive to be the best I can be and try everyday to be better than the day before.

All specialties of medicine and surgery have their value and demand. What I wanted was, not only to make a difference, but also personally feel satisfied. My discontent and dissatisfaction grew with each passing day. I felt as if I had missed my exit on the career highway because I was distracted by the dazzling lights in the distance. As I got closer, I realized it was nothing but construction vehicles and work lights. The only thing I wanted at this point was an opportunity for a quick U-turn, so that I could get where I should have gone in the first place.

It took me a couple more weeks to conger up the courage for the next step. I wanted a U-turn and that is what I was asking my residency director for. He could not understand where I was coming from and kept insisting that I would make a good surgeon, completely missing the point that I would have made an unhappy surgeon.

Finally I convinced the director that I would leave surgery no matter what and they gave in. I was lucky; I got good references and was accepted right away at the Wayne State University residency training program in medicine. Though located in a rough part of inner Detroit, and buried in snow nearly half the year, Detroit Receiving and Harper Hospitals made an exceptional training institution, one of the best in the country. Ignoring the drawbacks of the weather and the whereabouts, I was finally happy. Still working too many hours, I stayed frequently on call. I was just as poor and just as cold as I was back in New York but I knew my patients. I knew their personal and family history, and their social circumstances. I knew the intensity and nature of their pain and what relieved it. Now, going to bed in a different basement, I usually felt satisfied because when I made a difference in a patient's life, I usually knew how I did it and learned how to do it again.

So my learning to be a compassionate physician started from training in internal medicine and as everyone knows, the most common medical problem in our country is cardiovascular disease. This simply means dysfunction or disease of the heart and vessels. Since vessels are a part of every organ and tissue, the involvement of the vascular system affects everything. Understanding the cardiovascular system and keeping it in good health keeps the human body healthy. Essentially, health is the balance of the normal blood flow, maintaining electrolytes, hormones, oxygen, blood cells, stem cells and nutrient levels while disease is the disruption of the same.

Until recently most scientists thought that the heart cells can not replenish themselves, which means people die with the same heart they were born with. Dr. Piero Anversa of the Harvard Medical School first challenged this belief in 1987. He maintained that the heart muscle cells are definitely renewed and in fact renewed so fast that a person dying at the age of 80 has likely replaced the heart about four times over. This speed of renewal has never been confirmed, though in April 2009, Dr. Jonas Frisen at Karolinska Institute, Sweden, finally proved Dr Piero's basic assertion right. With the help of complex radioactivity calculations, he offered objective scientific evidence that about one percent of the heart muscle cells are replaced every year at age twenty five, and that rate gradually falls to less than half a percent per year by age seventy five. (18)

With this new discovery, came new possibilities. If the heart can generate new muscle cells, drugs can be developed that might accelerate this process and may open new approaches to treating heart disease. Since then, cardiac stem cells capable of long-term self-renewal and differentiation have also been identified, isolated and studied. (19)

In coronary heart disease there is reduction of the blood flow to the heart tissue. Reduced blood flow causes oxygen deprivation to the cells resulting in damage or death of these cells. This happens usually due to a blockage of the vessel supplying blood to a particular area of the heart. Muscle cells of the heart are not naturally replaced, so the left-over scar causes a functional decline of the heart as a pump. Depending on the size of the damage, this can lead to heart failure. The hope with the stem cell therapies is that once injected into the damaged area they will help repair the tissues, grow new vessels to promote blood flow and prevent scar formation that leads to impaired function and heart failure.

More than 50 randomized clinical trials have been published as of 2015, involving patients with a history of a heart attack or heart failure. A number of commercial biotechnology companies are spending millions of dollars on these trials and the results from many of these early-phase clinical trials have reported that adult stem cells are safe and effective in treating heart attack and heart failure. (20, 21)

Stem cell biology is experiencing rapid advances; in an attempt to capture the biggest market share the race for biotechnology companies is furious. Cardiac repair, through the use of regenerative medicine and adult stem cells, has been a considerable research focus over the last decade. Due to the high mortality and morbidity associated with coronary artery disease and heart failure, they remain a major target of these trials. (22, 23, 24)

Pre-clinical studies have clearly shown that the body mounts its own stem cell response in the event of a myocardial infarction (heart attack). Stem cell attractants such as vascular endothelial growth factor (VEGF) are observed in circulation following a heart attack. VEGF in turn promotes mobilization of bone marrow stem cells into the blood. This stem cell mobilization for myocardial repair seems to be a natural response of the body in case of tissue injury. (25, 26) It has also been established that the number of circulating stem cells in the blood is one of the best markers of cardiovascular health. Endothelial progenitor cells from bone marrow support the vascular endothelium lining and the number and function of these stem-like cells is inversely related to the cardiovascular risk. (27)

A reduction in these stem cells, therefore, increases the risk of adverse cardiovascular events while a higher number of circulating stem cells have a lower risk of a heart attack. (28) Studies show that if injected from an external source, the stem cells know how to find the site of cardiac tissue injury and home there. (29) Based on these and other pre-clinical studies, advanced clinical trials are now being planned. Cells derived from fat, skeletal muscles, peripheral blood, (30) bone marrow, (31, 32) umbilical cord blood, (33) and more recently, the heart itself, (34) have all been investigated as potential candidates for this treatment.

So far, cell therapies have shown a good safety profile but the proof of benefit has remained both variable and modest. So the potential clinical utility of this therapy remains experimental at this time. Last Cochrane review from 2012 stated "the results of this systematic review suggest that moderate improvement in global heart function is significant and is sustained long-term", but recommended larger trials. (35) The results of studies completed so far, show improvement of myocardial function, decrease in infarct size and reduction of major adverse cardiovascular events after treatment with stem cells. All these studies used adult stem cells from the patient (autologous).

The most promising results seem to be with the use of mesenchymal stem cells (MSCs) where evidence of improved cardiac function and better remodeling is found. (36) Preclinical studies have demonstrated that mesenchymal stem cells (MSCs) limit myocardial inflammation, cardiac cell death and promote new vessel formation (angiogenesis). (44) Clinical studies have also shown the ability of MSCs to inhibit post-infarct remodeling of the heart muscles, as well as block inflammatory processes in graft versus host reactions. (45, 46, 47)

Though initially believed to differentiate into new cardiomyocyte (heart cells), this was not the case in any of the cell types used. The benefit is more likely to be due to secretion of growth and other factors and stimulation of local cardiac stem cells. Research studies show mesenchymal stem cells to (1) inhibit myocardial inflammation (2) reduce cardiomyocytes apoptosis (3) and promote new vessel formation (angiogenesis). (37, 38, 39)

A number of companies are involved in testing these and other related ideas. Two major international phase III clinical trials have been recruiting patients. The first is a Belgian trial by Cardio 3 Biosciences, using its 'C-CURE' stem-cell therapy — a preparation of specially treated stem cells that are allegedly capable of developing into heart cells. This trial will include 480 patients with heart failure. The second is also a European trial called BAMI, and is testing standardized patient-derived stem cells. This study will include 3,000 patients with a history of recent heart attacks across Europe.

These are both Phase III trials. Please recall that this means the treatments have been accepted as safe and likely effective and this is the final phase before approval of their wide clinical use.

Several different methods have been employed in delivering these cells to the damaged hearts. These include injection in the area of the damaged heart, infusion in an artery supplying that area of the heart or directly into the blood stream. As yet no one has been able to establish:

1 - The best approach for delivery.
2 - The ideal stem cell candidate.
3 - The optimal dose, or
4 - The preferred time of administration after the injury.

All these questions remain unanswered.

Even the complete mechanism of the action of stem and progenitor cell regeneration remains uncertain. Several mechanisms have been proposed. There is evidence that infused stem cells induce paracrine cell-to-cell signaling, which may involve production of cytokines or other growth factors, that increase endogenous cellular repair and support increased collateral blood vessels. Only a very limited number of cells are noted to actually differentiate into heart cells. (40) It is likely that not one but a combination of these mechanisms are involved in the recovery process.

No one knows what the trials will show but there is a consensus that an ideal cardiac regenerative therapy would be a safe cell type, from an accessible source using the least invasive delivery technique. (41) The progress is rapid and

C-Cure and BAMI are not the only Phase III trials. At last count there were at least 15 more Phase III and many more Phase II clinical trials of stem cell products for cardiovascular disease progressing in hospitals around the world.

As yet the FDA or its European counterpart EMA (European Medicines Agency) has not authorized the clinical use of these stem cell products except in clinical trials. This has not, however, discouraged the commercial institutions operating outside the FDA/EMA jurisdiction to offer mesenchymal stem cell or umbilical cord cell therapies to patients with heart disease. For example, the Okyanos Heart Institute, in the Bahamas, uses mesenchymal stem cells derived from a patient for treatment of heart disease. These procedures remain without any solid evidence of efficacy.

The research for cardiac disease treatments is not limited to adult stem cells. Pre-clinical studies in animals, using embryonic stem cell-derived heart cells is also showing promise. They have already shown favorable effects of this treatment in small-animal models. (42) Now they are being tested in larger primates with equally positive results. In one of the studies non-human primate model of myocardial ischemia were treated with these cells and showed extensive muscular regeneration of the infarcted heart. Grafts were perfused by host vasculature, and electromechanical junctions between graft and host myocytes were present within 2 weeks of engraftment. (43)

Based on available data, cardiac cells or their precursors delivered to the heart after a heart attack or myocardial infarction can be potentially lifesaving. If the results of the Phase III clinical trials turn out to be as positive as the animal studies, it would transform the way we treat this group of patients. Would the winner be Adult Stem Cells, Embryonic Stem cells or induced Pluripotent Stem cells remains to be discovered? No matter the cell type, this field of medicine is slated to be the long term winner.

# Chapter 17

# CONCEPT TO CLINIC: Part II

The Role of Stem Cells in Neurological Diseases:

The HIV epidemic was at its peak in the 90s when I was going through my residency. Hospitals were full of sick and dying patients with AIDS. There was no shortage of gut-wrenching, heartbreaking tragedies in every hospital. Those patients made some of the saddest case studies. Talented young men in the prime of their lives and careers were attacked by a ruthless, sneaky and incurable invader.

The HIV didn't just ravage bodies; it also destroyed social lives and relationships. Parents were finding out for the first time they have a gay offspring and he is dying of AIDS. Families disowned their terminally ill sons on religious grounds, adamant that their congregation would never accept this "abomination". Friends left friends on their deathbed, concerned about what people might think if they found out about their friend with AIDS. In between admissions and transfusions, seizures and procedures, deaths and discharges, I saw new human tragedies unfolding around me day after day. After what I witnessed in that era, I am no longer surprised by any display of human selfishness. Why is it all about us? How anything affects us? How would it reflect on us? How would we be perceived? It is about our views, our beliefs, and our perceptions, no matter how it affects anyone else.

One winter evening while on call, I was preparing the next day's discharges and looking outside the window at miles of fresh snow reflecting the red glow of the setting sun. I heard a sobbing noise from one of the rooms. I knew the patient; Jessie, a 26 year old architect, admitted for shortness of breath, brought in by his boyfriend the night before. He was now emaciated and pale, with sunken eyes; though his bone structure, thick head of hair and big brown eyes told the story of a handsome face. He had a serious pneumocystis lung infection, common in advanced AIDS patients.

As I approached the room, I saw his boyfriend standing in the doorway crying. At first blush I thought the inevitable had happened, but I had heard no "code blue" and there was no medical staff around. Then I saw Jessie, who was awkwardly leaning forward from his pillow with the oxygen mask pulled off his face. With gasping breaths and eliding words he was making feeble attempts to yell at his father. It took me a minute to figure out the situation. Apparently, his father and brother had demanded that Jessie's boyfriend must leave if the family was to come visit him in the hospital. Clearly it had infuriated Jessie.

There are some words that never leave you; Jessie's rant that day was those sorts of words. Perspiring from exhaustion and fever, with heaving breaths, and in broken sentences, Jessie said, "My friend…..loves me ……..cares for me…stays up for me with no demands and no conditions………and you put conditions on your visit?......You don't need to disown me….I disown you…..I disown your world……..I disown……."

God knows what more Jessie wanted to say but the cough did not let him finish. I stepped up and replaced his oxygen mask, noticed his dropping oxygen level and increased the flow of oxygen; Jessie fell back in bed from exhaustion. I looked at his drawn, pinched, appearance and the dusky gray color of his face, ear lobes turned out, and the skin of his forehead parched and rough, muscles around the mouth completely relaxed; visible signs of his departure had arrived. His partner sat next to him and stroked his silky hair wet with sweat. Sometime during this commotion, his brother and father had left.

That was a life changing day for all involved. Jessie left this cruel world and passed on. His partner held Jessie's belongings close to his chest and left the hospital, with eyes full of pain and tears, and I sat down next to Gloria at the nurse's station, emotionally exhausted. Gloria was our wise, social worker, a motherly figure who I respected like a mentor. She patted my back with loving thumps, and then out of the blue she said, "You should become a physiatrist." I looked at her in surprise, "You know…..a rehabilitation specialist?" She must have seen…"?" written all over my face and elaborated, "Child, you will make a good physiatrist, because you have brains and you have compassion."

I was considering cardiology as my career option and at that time knew little about the evolving field of physical medicine and rehabilitation. Physiatry takes a comprehensive approach to managing chronic illnesses and disabilities. It is a specialty about the quality of life and getting people with illnesses, pain or injuries back on their feet with the help of all the medical treatments, practical methods and modern technology. On Gloria's encouragement, I opted to do a month of elective training at the Michigan Institute of Rehabilitation which happened to be conveniently next door to my hospital. My first day of that rotation, working with Dr. Steven Hinderer, I fell in love with the speciality. Here was a place where I could apply all my medical knowledge and compassion, manage all sorts of chronic diseases, do procedures to relieve pain, spasticity, deformity, and make people healthier and more functional with the help of therapists and equipment. Not only adding years to life, but also adding life to years.

That night I spent with Jessie and Gloria put me on the path I have been happily progressing along for over 15 years. I give thanks to everyone who helped me choose physiatry as my field of specialization. I later got accepted at the University of Texas South Western Medical Centre at Dallas. There I did my residency training in Rehabilitation Medicine, followed by advance trainings in Pain Management and later Regenerative Medicine. I enjoyed my years of training in orthopaedics, trauma, burns, spinal cord and brain injury care, stroke management and a long list of other chronic, disabling and painful conditions.

I have always felt close to my patients and though I am very fortunate not to suffer from any of the diseases or disabilities I treat, I know a thing or two about them. What you will read in the following passages is not just physiology, pathology and scientific facts. These are everyday facts of life for millions of people, who suffer from Parkinson's, or Alzheimer's, or Multiple Sclerosis, or any of the thousands of other diseases that ail humanity.

As rewarding as it is to help an elderly stroke victim get back on her feet, or a paralysed teenager play basketball again, even if from a wheelchair, or to see an army veteran with an amputation run on an artificial leg. It still leaves my heart aching with a wish that I could return them their pre-injury life. That is why I am so passionate about regenerative medicine, about stem cells, about hope, and chances and brighter possibilities for all those who need it…..who need it today. Let us look at some real possibilities.

## STEM CELL & NEUROLOGICAL DISEASES:

Since ancient times, the curiosity in one human brain has resulted in the exploration of another human brain; I mean literally. Healers in primitive days experimented on brains of prisoners and epilepsy sufferers. They learned and documented their findings in their treatise. It appears that the study of neurology dates back to prehistoric times and involved the opening of many heads. Over the centuries, it evolved from an observational science to a systematic way of approaching the nervous system and its affliction.

Hippocrates declared that epilepsy has a natural, not a supernatural cause. Aristotle described the meninges, cerebrum and the cerebellum. Sumerian illustrations show paraplegia caused by physical trauma, and ancient Egyptian treatise contains descriptions and treatment of various neurological injuries. Despite millennia of learning, neurological diseases remain some of the most debilitating, least understood, and hardest to treat conditions in medicine. Neurological diseases can be classified into degenerative, infectious, genetic, auto-immune, vascular and traumatic. The neurodegenerative group alone has too many members to be listed here, so we will look only at some of the common ones.

## ALZHEIMER'S DISEASE:

Alzheimer's disease is usually a disease of aging though one rare variant manifests earlier in life. Eventhough it was first described in 1906 by a German psychologist, Alois Alzheimer, the exact cause of this disease is still not well unerstood. (1)

There are several features of the disease that are suspect, including:

1 - Decreased connections and transmission between neurons,
2 - Formation of plaques in the brain made of amyloid protein that harden and choke the neurons,
3 - Abnormal Tau protein accumulation inside the neurons, which jumble up the nutritional microtubules creating a mesh of filaments known as the tau tangles,
4 - Damage to the insulating myelin sheath of the conducting neurons.

Regardless of its etiology Alzheimer's disease remains the most common cause of dementia, which is irreversible with current treatments. It is a slowly progressive brain disease that begins well before clinical symptoms emerge. The damage and death of neurons eventually impairs the ability to carry out even the basic bodily functions such as walking and swallowing.

Millions of Americans have Alzheimer's disease, and this number is expected to grow each year as the size and proportion of the population, aged 65 and older, continues to increase. An estimated 5.2 million Americans suffer form Alzheimer's disease. One in nine people aged 65 and older (11 %) have Alzheimer's disease. That number increases to about one out of three for people aged 85 and older. (2)

A healthy adult brain has about 100 billion neurons, each with long, branching extensions. In a normal brain the communication takes place at the junctions between neurons, called synapses. Through these synapses, information flows from one neuron to another by the process of neurotransmission. This information flows in the form of tiny bursts of chemicals, released by a conducting neuron and detected by a receiving neuron. A healthy adult brain contains about 100 trillion synapses. They allow signals to travel rapidly through the brain's circuits, creating the basis of memories, thoughts, sensations, emotions, movements and skills.

All information entering (sensory), or leaving (motor) the nervous system, is dependent on synaptic connections. There is a large variety of neurons involved in information relay within the nervous system. Different types of neurons use different transmitters at their synapses. For instance, motor neurons to the muscles, utilize neurotransmitter acetylcholine at the nerve muscle junction. The sympathetic transmission for a fight or flight response which causes goose bumps, an increased heart rate, and the dilation of pupils, uses adrenalin. Whereas the coordination of motor activities deep inside the brain controlled at the basal ganglia, involves the neurotransmitter Dopamine.

Besides being used at the nerve muscle junction, acetylcholine is also a widely used neurotransmitter in the brain. Acetylcholine is deficient in an Alzheimer's brain; therefore information transfer at synapses begins to fail, the number of synapses declines, and neurons eventually die. The current mode of treatment uses medications to increase this neurotransmitter, either by stimulating its production, or slowing its degradation. In both cases the effect is limited and benefit, transient, and partial.

There are no drugs that delay or halt the loss of neurons. No one has yet been able to determine the underlying cause for the development and progression of this devastating disease. What comes first… the plaques, the tangles, the decreased neurotransmitter, or the myelin damage? And which comes later as the consequence of the primary pathology? Until these questions are unequivocally answered, the chance of success in treating Alzheimer's remains rather bleak. Since there is no diagnostic test for Alzheimer's, the diagnosis is one of exclusion of other conditions, and confirmation only after a brain biopsy, usually at autopsy.

Another problem is the difficulty in creating animal models of this disease to study and test prospective treatments. Evolution of iPS cells that can be modified into brain cells is allowing the researchers a better chance to study the pathology and the stages of disease progression. Scientists have recently used iPS technology to grow neurons in the lab that show some of the key features of Alzheimer's disease. This approach holds great promise because it will allow better understanding, and may eventually help cure Alzheimer's disease.

Stem cells are an active area of research for Alzheimer's disease. Animal studies have shown initial promise, but this field of study is riddled with challenges. (3) Scientists are concerned that the brain may lack the ability to integrate new neurons properly once Alzheimer's has taken hold. Another concern is the damage to transplanted stem cells by the abnormal amyloid and tau proteins in the brain. This may mean only a temporary effect, if any.

Another approach to stem cell therapies is their use to deliver healing proteins called neurotrophins to the diseased brain. A healthy brain produces neurotrophins which support the growth and survival of neurons; their production is low in Alzheimer's. Neural stem cells that produce neurotrophins have shown memory improvement in animal models, human trials are now being considered. No proven, safe and effective stem cell treatment for this disease is yet available. More of the stem cell technology is currently being used to carry out rigorous studies on the causes and effects of Alzheimer's disease, rather than their direct use for cell-based therapies. (4, 5, 6)

PARKINSON'S DISEASE:

Parkinson's disease is a progressive neurodegenerative disorder characterized by tremors, rigidity, difficulty initiating movement and increasing problems with balance, gait and posture. According to the Parkinson's disease Foundation, Parkinson's disease affects about 1 million people in the US. Approximately 60,000 individuals are diagnosed with Parkinson's disease each year. It is the second most common neurodegenerative disease after Alzheimer's. A vast majority of Parkinson's cases occur sporadically, only 10% -15% of cases are hereditary. Less than 20% of cases affect people below the age of 50, the incidence increases after the age of 60. (7)

Although we know that people with Parkinson's have deficiency of the crucial neurotransmitter Dopamine in the neurons that control coordination of movements; the exact cause of Parkinson's disease remains a mystery. (8) Most drug therapies for Parkinson's only ameliorate the disease symptoms. It has long been known that when dopamine is reintroduced into the nervous system of animal or human patients, the symptoms of Parkinson's significantly improve. Since many symptoms are attributed to lack of dopamine, most treatments are geared towards its replacement.

Synthetic dopamine was developed in 1910, however, the protective blood brain barrier does not allow such large molecules to cross; therefore its size remained a challenge in its delivery to the brain. Dopamine precursors that can cross the blood brain barrier or smaller dopamine-like molecules are therefore used for treatment instead. (9)

None of these treatments are optimal, they all carry side effects and they work only for a few short years. Since we do not know how or why specific nerve cells die in the brains of Parkinson's patients, it is difficult to devise successful treatment. With the advent of iPS cell models of Parkinson's disease, researchers will be able to screen drugs more efficiently than possible with currently available animal models.

There is currently no cure for Parkinson's and we do not yet know its exact cause. Oral medications, supportive therapies and deep brain stimulation have all been used for treatment with limited success. Using stem cells to treat Parkinson's has become a realistic possibility in recent years. Replacing the lost dopamine-producing nerve cells with new, healthy cell transplant, offers exciting hope as a future cure for Parkinson's. (10)

Other treatment approaches are also being explored. An Australasian biotechnology company called, Living Cell Technologies (LCT) has developed a new product, NTCELL® that uses an alginate coated capsule containing clusters of neonatal porcine cells. After transplantation NTCELL® functions as a biological factory producing nerve growth factors to promote new central nervous system growth and repairs nerve degeneration. It is now in Phase I/IIa clinical trial in New Zealand for the treatment of Parkinson's disease. This product is purported to have other potential indications such as Huntington's, Alzheimer's and motor neuron diseases.

The most rational and promising approach, however, has been to treat Parkinson's by replacing damaged brain cells with new functional cells. Numerous animal experiments have provided evidence that implanted fetal neurons can replace dead neurons, form synapses and produce dopamine. Based on these results, centers around the globe attempted this procedure in humans with variable success. Lund University hospital in Sweden was one of the first centers to successfully treat Parkinson's with neural grafts from human fetal tissue. Of the patients treated worldwide with fetal dopamine-producing cell implants, most saw their symptoms improve markedly. Results over the last two decades, from these small trials indicate that patients can improve substantially with this treatment. (11) Recent reports also indicate that these implanted neurons survive in the patient's brain for more than a decade. (12)

However, because the source of the tissue is aborted fetuses, there are significant legal and ethical issues. To overcome these ethical and legal barriers, Dr. Michel Levesque, at Cedars-Sinai Medical Center and UCLA, for the last several years, has been using dopamine-secreting neurons derived from the patient's own brain stem cells. After growing these adult stem cells in the lab, they are transplanted back into that patient's brain. Most of his patients report significant reduction of the symptoms of Parkinson's disease. Adult stem cell therapy, therefore, offers the first of its kind treatment for Parkinson's which effectively reverses the progression of the disease. (13)

Dr. Levesque at UCLA, the researchers at Harvard Stem Cell Institute and many others around the globe are diligently working on improving this technique and trying to bring it into common practice. Additionally, other centers are working on iPS cells for similar applications which are now moving into clinical trials.

MULTIPLE SCLEROSIS:

Multiple Sclerosis (MS) or multiple scars (sclera = scar) has a well-documented history. The scar like plaques formed in the central nervous system gave MS its name. Symptoms consistent with the diagnosis of multiple sclerosis have been described since the 1300s. It is more common among people of northern European descent.

Factors such as modern diet, toxic exposure, vitamin D deficiency, and viral exposure have all been attributed as likely causes. Though not a hereditary disease, genetic variations have been shown to increase the risk of MS. (14) Environmental factors are also implicated. Several studies show that people who move to a different region of the world, before the age of 15 acquire the new region's risk to MS. However, if migration occurs after the age of 15, they retain their home country's risk. (15)

The real cause is probably a combination of both genetic and environmental factors. While the exact cause is not clear, MS is considered a disease of immune dysfunction, where the patient's immune cells attack the myelin sheaths that insulate the neurons. Just like an electrical wire with a damaged insulation, short circuits; neurons without their fatty myelin insulation cannot conduct electrical signals either. With sclerosis or plaques on the brain, spinal cord and nerves there is blocking of the impulse transmission, both sensory and motor transmission is impaired, producing neurological deficits.

Presentation of MS is quite variable and specific symptoms are determined by the locations of the sclerosis or plaques within the nervous system. Symptoms may include changes in sensation, muscle weakness, muscle spasms, difficulty with coordination and balance, fatigue, chronic pain, and bladder and bowel difficulties. Problems with speech, swallowing, and vision, can all be part of the presentation. (16)

There is no known cure for multiple sclerosis. Treatments attempt to improve functions after an attack, and prevent relapses. These treatments are only modestly favorable and have frequent adverse effects. Bone marrow transplants have been performed in patients who have aggressive non-responsive disease. The results of these experimental treatments are very promising but the procedure carries such a high mortality risk that it cannot be used as a routine procedure for every patient. Like many other neurodegenerative diseases, the hope is that stem cells may be able to reverse the carnage caused by this disease. These cells have the potential to facilitate repair of damaged nerve cells as well as appropriately modulate the abnormal immune response seen in MS patients.

Both in animal and human studies, Mesenchymal Stem Cells (MSCs), have shown immune regulatory properties which may stop the immune system from attacking the myelin sheath. MSC can be harvested from human umbilical cords besides other tissues. A growing body of evidence is proving mesenchymal stem cells to be more pluripotent than recognized before. More than 150 clinical trials around the world are currently testing the MSCs' ability to promote tissue repair in a variety of conditions such as osteoarthritis, diabetes, emphysema and stroke. (17) More than 20 of these trials are specifically for MS.

Experiments using MSCs to treat animal models of MS have been very encouraging. Phase I trials in Spain, Iran and China using adult MSCs to treat multiple sclerosis, reported no safety risks. Two FDA approved trials for

MS using MSCs harvested from a patient's own bone marrow were conducted here in the USA. One was at the Cleveland Clinic, infusing mesenchymal stem cells intravenously. The second conducted at the Tisch MS Research Center of New York, used mesenchymal stem cells that were first transformed in the laboratory into neural progenitor cells, and then injected into the spinal fluid. Their data on safety and dosing is also supportive of the procedure.

Alternate modes of stem cell treatment using Adult Hematopoietic Stem cells (HSC) transplant are also making gains. Recently, an Italian study showed sustained suppression of aggressive MS unresponsive to conventional therapies by using HSCs. Sustained clinical improvement, especially in the relapsing–remitting phase of the disease was reported. (18)

Besides the above Italian study, a Chinese study reaffirmed the above findings in its 2012 trial concluding, "Adult Hematopoietic SC transplant is a feasible treatment for severe MS and its long-term efficacy is favorable".(19) Another study concluded, "High-dose immunosuppressive therapy with autologous hematopoietic stem cell transplantation (AHSCT) is a promising approach to multiple sclerosis (MS) treatment." (20)

Richard Burt, MD, at Northwestern University is now running an international, randomized, open-labeled and partially-blinded trial, "Stem Cell Therapy for Patients with Multiple Sclerosis Failing Alternate Approved Therapy- a Randomized Study", *ClinicalTrials.gov Identifier: NCT00273364*. Additional phase II and phase III trials are also underway in other parts of the world. Nearly 1000 patients so far have received autologous HSC transplants for MS around the world and 2-year and 5-year follow up data is starting to come in. Results are not yet conclusive and larger multi-center randomized, double blind studies are recommended. Doctors and patients alike are keeping their fingers crossed for positive outcomes.

## AMYOTROPIC LATERAL SCLEROSIS (ALS)

There are two major types of cells in the brain, one that everyone knows are the quintessential brain cells or the neurons which transmit sensory and motor impulses. The other, just as important cells are the glial or the supporting cells. We have 50 times more glial cells than neurons in our brains. Glial cells are present throughout the brain providing infrastructure and support to the neurons. They also serve as the cleaning crew and nutrient supplier. Major types of glial cells in the brain are the Oligodendrocytes and the Astrocytes. Some diseases of the brain affect both these cell types; ALS is one of these diseases.

ALS, better known as Lou Gehrig's disease, is named after the famous American baseball player who suffered from the disease that ended his career and later his life. It is another degenerative and disabling central nervous disease which is rapidly progressive and fatal and which attacks the nerve cells (neurons) that control all the voluntary muscles in the body. Their job is to relay signals from the brain and spinal cord to the muscles in order to control movement. Since these neurons control motor functions, they are also known as motor neurons; ALS is therefore classified as a motor neuron disease.

ALS is one of the most common neuromuscular diseases worldwide. It affects people of all races but is more common among white males, generally aged 60–69 years, though younger and older people also develop the disease. According to the ALS Association, as many as 30,000 Americans have the disease, and the incidence is increasing each year. Ninty to nintyfive percent of all ALS cases are random or sporadic not hereditary, therefore other family members are not considered to be at an increased risk. Only 5 to 10 percent ALS cases are inherited.

The familial form of ALS usually results from a mutation in the gene that encodes the enzyme superoxide dismutase-1 (SOD1). (21) This enzyme is a powerful antioxidant that protects the body from damage caused by free oxygen radicles. Therefore, in its absence, free radicle damage results in the disease. A mouse model with this enzyme deficiency displays an ALS like disease.

ALS causes weakness in a wide range of muscles resulting in disabilities due to the loss of strength and ability to move the arms and legs, and causes slurred or nasal speech. Regardless of the part of the body first affected by the disease, muscle weakness and atrophy eventually spread to other parts of the body as the disease progresses. When muscles in the diaphragm and chest wall fail, people lose the ability to breathe on their own. Most ALS deaths occur due to respiratory failure, usually within 5 years from the onset of symptoms. Physicist Stephen Hawking who has suffered from ALS for almost 50 years is among the rare 4% cases of ALS who survive past 10 years. The disease usually does not impair intelligence, or cognitive functions as evident in the case of Mr. Hawkins. ALS also does not affect the vision, hearing or perception of smell and taste. (22)

The cause of ALS is unknown. Likely candidates are the abnormal SOD1 enzyme, abnormal processing RNA, environmental factors such as exposure to toxic or infectious agents, as well as physical trauma or behavioral and occupational factors. More recently there have been indications that rather than the primary defect being in the neuron itself it may be the surrounding glial cells that kill the motor neuron.

The diagnosis is based on patient history, good clinical and neurological exams, confirmed with the help of electro-diagnostic testing which uses the evaluation of the muscle's electrical signals to study the health or disease status of the muscle fibers. ALS has no known cure. FDA did approve a drug treatment— riluzole (Rilutek)—in 1995, which is reported to reduce motor neuron damage by decreasing the release of glutamate, (23) however, it prolongs survival only by a few months, without reducing the disability or reversing the damage to motor neurons, besides it is toxic to the liver. So essentially, there is no real treatment for the disease.

Laboratory studies suggest that certain types of stem cells may be effective for ALS treatment. Researchers have already conducted pre-clinical studies on mice using transplanted mesenchymal stem cells or neural progenitor cells in animals with ALS like neuron damage. These experimental, animal models showed a slowing of the motor neuron loss, and an improved lifespan. Human neural progenitor cell derived growth factor is also shown to help regrow motor neurons in rats. In addition, research in humans has shown that it is possible to transplant these engineered cells safely into the human spinal cord.

The biotechnology company, Neuralstem, initiated the first FDA-approved stem cell trial for ALS in January 2010 at Emory University. Based on this phase I trial data, Neuralstem cells were deemed to be safe, with no adverse reactions related either to cells or surgical techniques. The Phase II trials were approved by the FDA in April 2013 - and were completed in July of 2014, after final surgeries, which involved injections of human spinal cord stem cells into the diseased cord. The results so far show definite improvement, but only in patients in an earlier stage of the disease. (24, 25)

Stem cells clearly hold promise for a cure or remission in ALS and progress is being made, especially with the Neuralstem trial. It is, however, not the only company chasing the ALS cure. In June 2014, Brainstorm-Cell Therapeutics launched a phase II clinical trial in the United States. The participating clinical centres are the Massachusetts General Hospital, the Universityof Massachusetts Memorial Hospital, and the Mayo Clinic. It is a phase II, multi-center, randomized, double blind, placebo-controlled study using its product NurOwn™, to evaluate the safety and efficacy of autologous transplantation of neurotropic factor secreting Mesenchymal Stem Cells in 48 patients with ALS. *ClinicalTrials.gov Identifier:NCT02017912*. (26)

A second phase II NurOwn™ trial is running at Hadassah Medical Organization in Israel. *ClinicalTrials.gov Identifier:NCT01777646*. (27) Yet another ALS stem cell trial is currently enrolling 200 patients in India at the Neurogen Brain and Spine Institute to study the effect of autologous bone marrow mononuclear cells on Amyotrophic Lateral Sclerosis patients *ClinicalTrials.gov ID: NCT02242071*. A comprehensive list of ALS trials is available at http://www.als.net/ALS-Research/ALS-Clinical-Trials

STROKE:

Hippocrates is credited as the first physician to have recognized stroke, more than 2400 years ago. In one of his aphorisms, Hippocrates stated, "Unaccustomed attacks of numbness and anesthesia are signs of impending apoplexy". Stroke was known as apoplexy (struck down by violence) in Greek, describing a sudden collapse, a loss of consciousness, and paralysis. (28)

It was not until the 1600s, that a vascular cause of stroke was established. In 1928, stroke was classified, based on the vascular pathology, and was named Cerebral Vascular Accident (CVA) and more recently "Brain Attack", since it is also caused by a lack of blood supply to the brain; much like a heart attack is caused by a lack of blood supply to the heart.

Stroke is a leading cause of death and the most common cause of physical disability in adults, for which there is no effective treatment. Strokes happen when blood flow to the brain stops. Brain cells begin to die within minutes. (29) There are two kinds of stroke. Ischemic stroke, the more common kind, is caused by a blood clot that blocks a blood vessel in the brain. The other kind is hemorrhagic stroke, which is caused by the rupture of a blood vessel which results in bleeding within the brain. Both types cause brain cell (neuronal and glial) damage and death that remain irreparable with existing therapies. The loss of neurons in the cerebral cortex is a major cause of stroke-induced neurological deficits. Stroke can cause permanent motor impairment, speech deficits, and behavioral incapacity.

Therapeutic options for a stroke are limited; various approaches to protect brain function and prevent further ischemic damage have remained unsuccessful. A large proportion of stroke survivors, therefore, live with severe disabilities, associated with a high personal and financial cost. Clot dissolving (Thrombolytic) therapy is currently the only available stroke treatment, but it can only be offered to a small number of patients, and only within a short window of time. Once the damage is done, current treatment options do not offer any recovery in the brain itself, the natural plasticity of the brain does allow for the formation of new connections and some natural healing over time. However, rehabilitation and prevention of complications remains the mainstay of long-term management with limited functional recovery.

The brain does have two caches of stem cells (periventricular and hippocampus areas), but their number and activity is not enough to compensate the usual damage caused by a stroke. In recent years, there has been a wave of interest in these stem cell populations. Scientific research has provided information on how stem cells improve aspects of cellular and functional recovery following strokes in animal models. Based on these pre-clinical studies, stem cell transplantation has emerged as a promising new experimental treatment for stroke. (30)

Transplantation of Neural Stem Cells (NSCs), derived from human iPSCs in a stroke model, have shown that these NSCs which are the precursors of neurons and glia, survived and differentiated primarily into neurons. (31) A number of clinical trials have been undertaken to understand the mechanism of the action of these cellular therapies, their safety and efficacy. (32, 33, 34, 35, 36)

Additional studies are now underway. Cell replacement therapy, gene transfer, and selective repair of injured neural cells into diseased areas of the brain, are a rich area of research with new information pouring almost daily. Cell transplantation is an especially promising potential treatment for stroke recovery and multiple cell types have shown promise in stroke models. There is great potential for new therapeutic developments for diseases of the nervous system from several of these approaches. (37, 38, 39, 40)

The first North American trial of intra-parenchymal transplantation of bone marrow-derived cell therapy for chronic stroke patients recently published its results concluding that intra-parenchymal transplantation of human bone marrow-derived stromal cells in chronic stroke patients is safe, feasible, and shows a trend towards neurologic improvement. (41) Multiple other trials are underway attempting to answer lingering questions. How beneficial these treatments really are? What is the best type of stem cell for this indication? What dose and mode of administration of stem cells will produce best outcome? (42,43,44,45,46,47,48)

A recent study performed at the Imperial College NHS Trust, London, UK used intra-arterial injection of CD34+ stem cells for acute ischemic stroke. The procedure was well-tolerated with no significant adverse effects. All patients showed improvements in clinical functional scores, as well as reductions in lesion volume at 6-month follow-ups. All five people in this pilot study, who had suffered severe strokes, regained the power of speech, use of their arms and legs, as well as improved cognition after only six months post treatment. (49)

A newer approach to the cell replacement therapy is the use of iPS derived oligodendrocyte progenitor cells (OPCs), and neural progenitor cells (NPCs) for regenerative treatments. Human induced pluripotent stem cells (iPSCs) have extensive proliferation potential and the unique ability to produce any type of somatic cells. (50, 51) This new source of cells is expected to increase the rate at which we are getting close to a usable solution in the treatment of neurological diseases, including stroke. A number of questions remain regarding mechanisms by which these cells exert their neuro-protective effects. With a better understanding of how cell-based therapies ameliorate stroke injury a wealth of information and evidence supporting stem cell use is converging and is bound to help transition basic research into clinical applications. The future is promising, though for millions of people who are suffering from stroke and its related disability, answers cannot come soon enough.

# Chapter 18

# CONCEPT TO CLINIC: Part III

Stem Cells Healing Cartilage Bone and Joints

In 2009, while working in Australia, one day a veterinarian friend of mine, asked me to teach her how to do liposuction. I asked her, "On your husband"? She laughed and said, "Shhhh!" But she was serious. She wanted to do liposuction on dogs. But why? Apparently, many veterinarians started using stem cell treatments for animals more than a decade ago. These cells were derived from the animal's fat and my friend wanted to offer the benefits of this technology to her own furry patients.

Vet-Stem, Inc., a privately held company from San Diego, California was the first US Company to provide a fat-derived stem cell service for horses, dogs, cats, and some exotic animals in 2002. Vet-Stem developed therapies in veterinary medicine that utilize the natural healing properties inherent in all animal stem cells. According to the company's press releases, Vet-Stem holds exclusive licenses to over 50 patents including world-wide veterinary rights for use of adipose-derived stem cells. Over 10,000 animals, including more than 4000 horses, have been treated using Vet-Stem regenerative technology. The company is actively investigating stem cell therapies for immune-mediated and inflammatory diseases, as well as solid organ diseases. Data has so far been published in 11 peer-reviewed papers; this includes the first randomized, double blind, controlled, multicenter study of adipose-derived stem cells for chronic osteoarthritis in the canine hip joint. (1)

Vet-Stem cell procedures are used for the treatment of tendon and ligament injuries and have become the gold standard for performance horses with these injuries. The success rate in the follow-up studies is impressive and often makes news headlines. Greater than 75% of horses treated with Vet-Stem Cell therapy for tendon and ligament injuries are reported to return to their previous level of performance including competitive level sports. (2)

Vet-stem is not alone in this arena; a number of new companies are now operating in this space, including, Animal Cell Therapies, Inc., Nupsala Stem Cell Therapy, Penn Vet, and VetCell Bioscience Ltd. The last one is a Cambridge-based UK company that expands the Mesenchymal Stem Cells (MSC) outside the body before injecting them back. VetCell's own literature claims that it has pioneered a technique to affordably multiply equine mesenchymal stem cells from bone marrow. These stem cells can either be used immediately, or cryogenically preserved for future use. The cells are implanted into the core of the lesion, and the animal enters a controlled rehabilitation program to promote appropriate differentiation of the cells. Clinical and ultrasonographic improvement of the tendon is well-documented in treated animals.

VetCell has a sister company called MedCell which is providing treatment protocols and equipment for similar treatment in humans. The earliest studies in rats and rabbits, demonstrated both improved strength and quality of reparative tissue (collagen), with the use of BM-derived MSCs. (3, 4) Success with animal experience has resulted in similar procedures being tested in humans. A sample of fat is removed from the patient that is spun and washed with saline; stem cells are then separated in a syringe for injection into the injury site. Sadly though, animals have had years of benefit from these treatments while humans faced a variety of restrictions against the use of their stem cells for their own health improvement. The animal studies did allow a platform to build on, and use this preclinical data to start clinical trials in humans.

Fat-derived stem cells are a known source of tissue regeneration and demonstrate the potential of differentiation into tendon cells in vitro and in animals. (5) These are the same Mesenchymal stem cells (MSC) that we have talked about in several other disease chapters; your own cells, taken from fat or marrow, separated and injected into a joint, muscle or ligament. These have both, regenerative and the immunosuppressive properties. (6)

Fat is an obvious choice for extraction of these cells because it is usually in abundance, which any patient is happy to part with, and contains a surprisingly high number of stem cells. One gram of fat contains up to 1,000,000 MSCs. In comparison, the same amount of bone marrow has less than 1,000 MSCs. The large numbers and ready availability of MSCs in fat usually does not require expansion or a culture of the cells. When cells are extracted from fat, they contain a variety of stem and progenitor cells that normally lie hidden in the tissues. These include endothelial progenitor cells known to increase angiogenesis (new blood vessel formation) and other cells like macrophages that secrete anti-inflammatory cytokines. Most procedures utilize this entire mixture of cells along with the MSCs.

OSTEOARTHRITIS:

Osteoarthritis is an extremely common age-related degeneration of joints, more in the weight-bearing joints like the knee and the hip, but also the joints of the hand, shoulder, wrist and spine. It is a common source of pain and disability. This is a progressive condition with no cure, so obviously there is a great deal of interest in learning about the application of stem cells for repair and relief. Additionally, many moderately severe orthopedic injuries, such as rotator cuff tears, that undergo surgeries, may fail; therefore the possibility of stem cell application to either replace or enhance surgical benefits would be widely welcome. Other conditions that are often difficult to treat and are not amenable to surgery such as Achilles tendonitis, chronic tennis elbow inflammation, and plantar fasciitis, are also likely to respond to MSC treatments, based on animal experience, clinical trials are now progressing at centers around the globe.

More and more trials are moving into the human testing stage; a recent study published in September 2014 in the journal, "International Orthopedics", showed significant improvement in healing outcomes achieved by the use of bone marrow-derived MSC, as an adjunct therapy to standard care of rotator cuff repair. Furthermore, this study also showed a substantial improvement in the level of tendon integrity present at the ten-year milestone between the MSC-treated group and the control patients. These results support the use of bone marrow-derived MSC augmentation in rotator cuff repair, especially due to the enhanced rate of healing and the reduced number of re-tears observed over time in the MSC-treated patients. (7)

Cellular Biomedicine Group Inc. is a publicly traded company that is testing its fat-derived mesenchymal precursor cell called ReJoin™ for knee arthritis in humans. It is now in its Phase IIb trial to further evaluate its safety and efficacy. The six-month follow-up of the Phase IIa trial was completed in 2013 and confirmed that this therapy is safe, and showed an increase in cartilage volume as early as three months after the treatments.

Besides Cellular Biomedicine Group Inc. and MedCell Inc., their Australian counterpart, Regeneus, also offers commercial regenerative products HiQCell (for humans) and AdiCell (for animals). These are relatively simple procedures that use mesenchymal stem cells taken from the patient's own adipose (fat) tissue through mini liposuction. The adipose tissue is then processed into a cell suspension, which is injected into the injured tissue or arthritic joint for repair.

A second veterinary product by Regeneus, both for canine and equine fields, is called Cryoshot. Unlike AdiCell, Cryoshot is an allogenic product (derived from another person or animal). The advantage of allogenic products is that they are available off the shelf and ready to use right away in contrast to autologous that have to be removed from the animal, and need to be processed and prepared before use. Safety and efficacy studies show it to be a safe treatment with variable benefits in different patients. Regeneus has another technology platform, based on cytokine secretions from stem cells rather than cells themselves. This platform has potential applications in the healing of wounds, burns, acne or other skin conditions that can be treated with a cream.

Products such as HiQcell, STEMPRO®, ATCC®, MesenCult™ AdiStem Ltd., MyCells®, and dozens of other similar products, are already in use in many countries including Australia, the USA and several EU member countries. These companies provide simple-to-use kits, where the liposuctioned fat or aspirated bone marrow can be processed in the doctor's office. This generally takes 1-2 hours and is injected back into the patient at that same visit.

Skeptics assert that the clinical use of stem cells pushed by the commercial companies is behind the curve of the research proof. However, these procedures are based on ample basic and clinical studies and have repeatedly passed the safety test when practiced in a safe environment and competent hands.

My personal experience with hundreds of patients, shared experience of peers in the field, published and presented data, as well as recent studies, all show significant improvement in properly-selected patients with appropriate diagnosis. Competent providers like Dr. Christopher J. Centeno in Colorado, USA; Dr. Peter Lewis in Melbourne, Australia, Professor Jaroslav Michalek at Cellthera in Brno, Czech Republic, and several others have been consistently showing reproducible benifits in properly selected patients and have data to prove it. Difficulty arises when some providers attempt to treat everyone and everything with stem cells. The fact is that nothing works for everything; so when you hear implausible claims of cures for everything from flu to AIDS; exercise caution.

A review of available literature over the last decade, related to the use of stem cells in sports injuries, shows the potential for clinical efficacy, based on the data available from basic science and animal studies. (8,9,10,11,12). There are now several studies illustrating the potential for the use of stem cells, not only in tendon repair, but also their use in other tissue engineering applications. The use of stem cells is becoming a promising treatment in the armamentarium of the physician or surgeon in the field of musculoskeletal medicine. (13)

An impressive amount of work is going on around the world, mainly in Korea, China, Australia and the EU. Unfortunately, in the USA, significant regulatory hurdles have hampered progress. Current Food and Drug Administration (FDA) regulations prohibit any expansion or manipulation of the stem cells, unless the product is administered under an investigational new drug application. This means an investment of millions of dollars, thousands of pages of regulatory paperwork, and years of testing. Other countries, where the regulatory structure is more sensible and less restrictive, are investigating a variety of new methods. The following is an account of some of the most recent work.

Elderly patients treated with fat-derived stem cells for knee osteoarthritis, all showed significant improvement in clinical outcomes. They significantly improved at 1 year, and even more at 2-year follow-ups. The study concluded that fat-derived stem cell therapy for elderly patients with knee OA is effective in cartilage healing, reducing pain, and improving function. (14)

Osteonecrosis or bone death in the hip joint is an established complication of trauma, excessive alcohol consumption, HIV infection or prolonged steroid use. The only effective treatment is hip replacement surgery. The efficacy and safety of autologous bone marrow mesenchymal stem cell (BMMSC) was tested with injections into the medial circumflex femoral artery for the treatment of hip osteonecrosis. This study from 2013 showed a relief of symptoms, an improvement of hip function and a delay in the progression of bone death. This work demonstrated that this method of autologous BMMSC perfusion is a safe, effective and minimally invasive treatment strategy for early-stage osteonecrosis of the femoral head. (15)

A South Korean proof-of-concept trial published in May 2014, reported that direct injection of autologous adipose-derived culture-expanded MSCs into osteoarthritic knees improved pain and knee function, with no treatment-related adverse events. A 6-month MRI evaluation showed regenerated articular cartilage in the MSC group as measured by cartilage volume and patients showed an improvement in clinical outcomes when compared with control groups. A second Korean trial used intra-articular injection of adipose-derived stem cells in 30 older patients with knee osteoarthritis. At two-year follow-ups patients had significantly improved pain and function. Only five patients demonstrated worsening of symptoms but none underwent total knee replacement during the study period. (16)

Meniscus damage due to injury or age-related degeneration is a common source of knee pain and functional impairment. More and more studies are reporting that intra-articular injection of stem cells into the knee is effective in promoting healing after meniscal surgery. In a multicenter American study of an expanded allogeneic MSC product, recently published in the "Journal of Bone and Joint Surgery", reported that patients who received higher or lower doses of MSC gel, compared to hyaluronic acid (HA) alone, showed favorable results in 57 patients who had undergone partial meniscectomy. A follow up MRI at 1 year showed meniscal regeneration and increased meniscal volume in some participants. Both groups who received MSC had statistically significant improvements in pain compared with those receiving hyaluronic acid alone. (17)

The knee is not the only joint being studied. In a recent case series of 20 patients at high risk for non union who underwent ankle fusion, Hyer et al, used allograft cells with internal fixation surgery. Results showed that the allograft improved both the rate and speed of healing compared to traditional methods in high-risk patients. (18)

A Korean study on the ankle also recently published findings that using MSCs improved results in ankle procedures in patients at high risk for poor outcomes. They treated one group of ankle cartilage lesion patients with the traditional surgical approach and the other group with the same procedure plus injection of autologous MSCs derived from fat. Both groups had decreased pain and improved recovery scores, but the patients receiving stem cells had significantly greater improvement in their recovery scores and activity levels as well as shorter return-to-activity times. (19)

From research studies and experience in clinical practice, the safety of MSC in musculoskeletal injuries, with or without surgery, is no longer in question; some level of benefit has also been established; the extent of this benefit is more of the debate at this point. More robust human clinical trials are on the way; such clinical trials are necessary to clarify conclusive benefits as well as the methodology of treatment. Hopefully with relaxation of restrictions and more frequent use of autologous stem cells in this space, answers will be forthcoming.

Despite the paucity of high level scientific literature on this subject there is no shortage of anecdotal case reports. A part of the reason why stem cell use in musculoskeletal injuries has gotten more press than other applications has to do with the frequent reports of high-profile athletes undergoing stem cell procedures. More than 200 NFL players have reportedly undergone such treatments, some publicly acknowledging the treatment while others keeping it private. I believe those days are not far when one will not have to be a sports icon to take advantage of these treatments.

*Why do you stay in prison, when the door is so wide open?*
*- Rumi*

# Chapter 19

# CONCEPT TO CLINIC: Part IV

Role of Stem Cells in Diseases of the Liver and Pancreas:

## LIVER

I recall watching old movies where every dying person bled from their mouth. That may have been for theatrics, but real life patients with liver failure do die bleeding from all orifices. It is a serious, often fatal, and unfortunately far too common of a condition. Most common causes are excessive alcohol use and chronic hepatitis infection. The reason for the bleeding is the lack of coagulation proteins produced in the liver. It is only one of the hundreds of vital functions that the liver performs every day.

Besides its vital role in the detoxification of blood; the synthesis of proteins, cholesterol, bile salts and vitamins; storing a variety of essential nutrients, and playing an essential role in controlling blood glucose, the human liver is a model of regeneration. It is well-known that mature liver cells can duplicate in response to injury. Liver regeneration has been recognized for ages, dating all the way back to Prometheus in ancient Greek mythology. Even if three-quarters of a liver is surgically removed, it has enough regenerative ability to return to normal functions by duplication of its cells. (1)

The normal liver regenerates through division of mature liver cells (hepatocytes). This capacity, however, is lost in chronic liver diseases. A backup repair system in the liver consists of progenitor liver cells (semi-differentiated stem cells), called oval cells. In addition, multiple scientific reports have demonstrated that bone marrow cells can also give rise to a variety of hepatic cell types. Hence there are several modes of liver regeneration. (2)

The end-stage liver disease is a serious health problem, and liver transplantation is currently the only effective therapy. However, donor shortage, operative damage, and the risk of rejection, account for the growing interest in regenerative medicine. Scientists have been searching for the optimal source of stem cells that can generate large amounts of hepatocytes for bio-artificial livers or for the injection into the patient, to repair the diseased organ. Based on research reports, under proper experimental conditions, adult, embryonic and fetal stem cells are all capable of differentiation into hepatocytes. In the future, stem cell-derived hepatocytes will likely be employed as, "bridge therapy" for patients with liver failure awaiting transplantation, or for independently recovering liver function. Intrahepatic injection of stem cell-derived hepatocytes might also be useful in patients with acute liver failure. (3)

The latest research by Harvard scientists has provided new evidence that it is possible to repair a chronically diseased liver by reprogramming liver cells. Essentially it means that appropriate signaling can turn back the clock in mature liver cells and make them stem cell-like, to regenerate a diseased liver. This suggests another mode of regeneration at work which possibly helps repair more persistent liver damage, as in chronic diseases. (4)

Based on this research, it may be possible to grow liver progenitor cells in mass quantities in a laboratory for cell transplants, avoiding the need for a whole organ transplant. Clinicians have been trying liver cell transplantation for metabolic liver diseases since the 90s. However, these attempts have failed, likely because the cells came from discarded livers. The new mechanism of reprogrammed cells may finally lead to success, but remains to be seen in human trials.

Due to the prevalence of liver disease, and the shortage of donors, the Mayo Clinic surgeons have been performing living donor liver transplants for over a decade. This procedure counts on the exceptional regenerative potential of liver tissue, where a portion of a living donor's liver is removed and used to replace a matching patient's diseased liver. After surgery, both livers regenerate back to normal size. Despite reassuring long term follow up of the live donors, it remains a risky procedure and better alternatives are constantly being sought.

In 2013, Japanese researchers from the Okohama City University used human skin-derived, induced pluripotent stem cells (iPSc) to form the three main types of liver cells. These hepatic endoderm cells, mesenchymal cells, and endothelial cells were mixed together to grow a liver. It was then transplanted into a mouse where it formed connections with the blood vessels and started functioning as normal liver tissue. Other scientists this year reported in the journal "Applied Materials & Interfaces", a new way to inject stem cells from tonsils into damaged livers for repair, and demonstrated improvement in function, all without surgery. (5)

Just like dialysis machines that clean the blood of patients with kidney failure, an artificial liver apparatus called Spheroid Reservoir Bio-artificial Liver, has been undergoing trials using pig liver cells. The future use of human cells in this apparatus is the focus of some research centers. Additionally, these mini livers may one day be used for drug testing or even for transplants. Current liver transplantation does not use patient-specific cells and requires immuno suppression. The advent of iPS derived liver cell transplant may drastically improve this complication as well.

Researchers are now attempting to grow a pancreas in the same fashion as the liver. Other Harvard scientists have discovered the signals that help stem cells decide whether to become liver or pancreas cell. This knowledge is helping scientists differentiate stem cells in the right direction. Though liver and pancreas are very different organs with hugely different functions, at the embryological level both have the same endodermal origin from the gut.

## PANCREAS:

Pan-Kreas, as known to the Greek, translates into "all flesh". Probably because of its position, it was thought to be a soft packing to protect the major vessels (Aristotle) or cushion the stomach (Galen). The pancreas is a solid gland, about 10-15 cm. long, located in the upper left abdomen, behind the stomach. It is surrounded by the small intestine, liver, and spleen. The pancreas is a dual-function gland, having features of both a larger exocrine component that produces digestive enzymes, and a smaller endocrine component that produces hormones. The most important and well known of these hormones is insulin.

Even though diabetes had been known and documented for just as long as the existance of pancreas, it was not until the late 19th century that the role of the pancreas in the development of diabetes was finally established. (6) Different cultures identified and reported diabetes differently. For example, the ancient Indians tested for diabetes by observing whether ants were attracted to a person's urine, and called the ailment "sweet urine disease". It has taken centuries to arrive at the current understanding and knowledge about the pancreas, and the search and discovery is ongoing. The most important endocrine function of the pancreas is the production of insulin, by its β-cells. The deficiency of insulin causes diabetes. The story of diabetes, however, is complex, with two distinct varieties.

**Diabetes, Type 1**: In this disease that manifests early in life, the body's immune system is misled into attacking and destroying its own insulin-producing β-cells of the pancreas. (7) The lack of insulin prevents regulation of blood sugar which rises out of control. The end result is the need of external insulin to manage the blood sugar levels in order to prevent complications.

**Diabetes, Type 2**: In this case the body cells develop resistance to the insulin later in life, impacted by body weight and an inactive life style. As a result, more and more insulin is required to regulate blood sugar levels. The constant demand on the pancreas for an ever-increasing amount of insulin eventually burns out the β-cells. (8) Once the pancreas loses its ability to produce adequate amounts of insulin, the blood sugar level starts rising. In the early stages of the disease, medications can help improve blood glucose but in the end, the need for external insulin to manage the blood sugar levels is inevitable.

Stem cells hold the promise to someday replace these dead insulin-producing cells. However, it is important to recognize that though in both types of diabetes the end result is lack of insulin, the underlying pathology is distinctly different. Implantation of new pancreatic cells alone will not solve the problem in either case.

In the case of Type 1 diabetes, any new pancreatic cells will be destroyed by the hyperactive immune system, so the immune system needs to be brought under control before donor cells or stem cell-derived pancreatic cells can be transplanted. In the case of Type 2 diabetes the peripheral resistance of the tissues to insulin needs to be addressed, otherwise any new pancreatic $\beta$-cells will soon burn out as well.

Islet transplantation from a postmortem pancreas has thus far provided a foundation for the next-generation cell-based therapeutics for diabetes. More than 50% of subjects treated with pancreas transplant from cadavers gained insulin independence 1 year post-transplantation without hypoglycemic episodes, with 20% remaining insulin therapy-free 5 years after transplantation. (9, 10)

However, the shortage of donor pancreas, the chances of rejection, and a 50% or higher failure rate has prompted search for better options. Recently all hopes have been pinned on stem cell cures and experience is amassing with multipotent mesenchymal stem cells. (11)

MSCs are being evaluated not only for their cellular differentiation into $\beta$-like cells but also for their potent anti-inflammatory and immune-suppressive effects. (12, 13) All cell types are being extensively reviewed to see which one fits the bill. These include mesenchymal, hematopoietic, induced pluripotent and pancreatic stem cells. (14, 15)

ViaCyte, Inc., a privately-held, regenerative medicine company, got FDA approval in August 2014 for Phase II clinical trial of its VC-01, in type-1 diabetes patients. ViaCyte will use VC-01, a stem cell-derived, encapsulated cell replacement therapy as a potential cure for type-1 diabetes. The 2-year trial will involve four to six testing sites, the first being at UC San Diego, which will recruit approximately 40 study participants. The advantage of encapsulated beta cells is that they can assess the patient's glucose level in the blood and secrete the correct amount of insulin, while their capsule barrier protects them from any attack by the autoimmune system.

While ViaCyte from west coast (UC San Diego), received its FDA approval to progress with its embryonic stem (ES) cell trial, a group of scientists from the east coast (Harvard University), led by Dr. Doug Melton, reported the successful development of mature beta cells, both from human ES cells and human induced pluripotent stem cells (iPSCs). They used these beta cells, derived from ES cells, to "cure" diabetes in their mouse-models. According to a company release, "Melton's final cells reliably respond to glucose and make insulin as needed". BetaLogics™ is yet another company that has reported similar pre-clinical success with ES cells for diabetes.

Despite notable progress, the clinical development of cell therapies using human embryonic stem cells continues to be surrounded by ethical concerns. Therefore, scientists have continued to follow all other avenues that may lead them to insulin-producing cells. Most of these trials are exploiting the properties of adult and induced pluripotent stem cells to provide both the cellular and the immune modulatory benefits.

A large multicenter trial in 11 of the States in the USA is being sponsored by an Australian company, Mesoblast™ This trial is also assessing the safety and effectiveness of donated cells (termed MPC-mesenchymal progenitor cells) in type 2 diabetes patients. The trial will recruit 60 participants with type 2 diabetes who have poor control of their disease with medications. The subjects will be monitored for complications and for changes in the control of their diabetes.

In other parts of the world, similar trials are being conducted using, embryonic, induced and adult stem cells. A trial is being conducted at the PLA Hospital in Sichuan province, China that aims to recruit a total of 60 subjects. The trial will use Adult Bone Marrow Stem Cells and is expected to run until December 2015. It is a phase I/II study for safety and efficacy. A similar Phase I/II trial in China is being conducted at the Peking University Aerospace Centre Hospital in Beijing and expects to enroll 500 patients.

In India trials are being conducted by the Post-Graduate Institute of Medical Research in Chandigarh, to compare different methods of delivering the patient's own bone marrow stem cells. A second trial at the same institute is investigating the efficacy of stem cells derived from the patient's own bone marrow in the treatment of type 2 diabetes. Mesenchymal stem cells are harvested from the patient's own bone marrow and expanded in the laboratory, before injecting them into the blood supply of the pancreas. Patients in a control group receive a placebo injection in exactly the same manner as the experimental group. This trial is expected to run till June 2015.

The new frontier is the Induced Pluripotent Stem Cells (iPSCs); their differentiation into functional $\beta$ cells is now well documented and provides the basis of new diagnostic and therapeutic applications. Both Type 1 and Type 2 diabetes-specific iPSCs have already been derived from patients. (16, 17, 18, 19) iPSC derived from healthy patients have shown the capability to generate insulin-producing cells and their autologous property is expected to prevent rejection in cell-based therapy for diabetes. (20, 21)

A variety of other approaches to treat diabetes were tested in the past with mixed results. Animal and clinical studies have now shown that moderate immunosuppression in type 1 DM can prevent further loss of insulin-producing cells. A clinical trial (Identifier: *NCT00315133*) in 2007 involving high-dose immunosuppression and autologous hematopoietic stem cell transplantation was performed with acceptable toxicity in a small number of newly diagnosed type 1 DM patients. The results showed that the beta cell function was increased in 13-14 patients with insulin-free episodes for an average of 16 months. (22) This, however, is a dangerous procedure with significant risks. Safer alternatives are constantly being sought. The immune modulation properties of Mesenchymal stem cells, as tested above, are now the focus of studies where safer methods of their introduction are being sought.

Despite promising results on several fronts, there remain challenges when using pluripotent stem cells:

- First is the ability to achieve reliable and efficient differentiation into insulin-producing islet-like cells.
- Second is to overcome the difficulty in generating insulin-producing cells that are glucose-responsive so that they do not just continue to produce insulin out of control causing hypoglycemia.
- Third is the challenge of protecting these cells from the immune attack so that they are not destroyed by the body.
- Fourth there always remains the risk of tumor formation whenever pluripotent cells are used.

After all of these challenges have been surmounted there will be the commercial challenge of providing proof of safety and efficacy to get the FDA approval. Finally, if approved, we actually may get to use them in real life.

The good news is that progress is being made on every one of these fronts and tangible results are expected soon. I cannot wait for the day when we are able to tap into the amazing potential of stem cells and people with diabetes won't have to live with daily insulin injections, the agony of high and low blood sugar, and the painful damage to their kidney, heart, brain, eyes and nerves.

*Cease looking for flowers; there blooms a garden in your own home.*
*~Rumi*

# Chapter 20

# STEM CELLS AND SPINAL CORD INJURY

*There is a life-force within your soul, seek that life.*
*There is a gem in the mountain of your body, seek that mine.*
*O traveler, if you are in search of that, don't look outside,*
*look inside yourself and seek to find.*
*~ Rumi*

**Clinical Trials and Financial Tribulation**

Every year, in the USA, about 12,000 people experience a spinal cord injury or SCI. Most often, it results from trauma. Approximately 3 million people around the world live with this devastating injury. SCI pathology is characterized by the loss or damage of neurons and their supporting cells called oligodendrocytes. The spinal cord extends down from the base of the brain and gives out a pair of nerves at each cervical, thoracic, lumbar and sacral region. These nerves supply muscles and skin, collecting and distributing neuronal messages to and from the brain.

Damage to this major conduction pathway disconnects part of the body below the level of injury, from the brain. This results in loss of muscle movement, sensation, and bowel / bladder control. Injury can be due to a knife or gunshot wound, a fall, a motor vehicle accident, sports or any other type of crush injury. The damage results from either the loss of nerve fibers or the glial cells that insulate these fibers. In a majority of SCI cases, there is contusion, rather than a complete severing of the nerve fibers. A spinal cord injury (SCI) damages both the gray matter (cell bodies) and the white matter (cell fibers) in the cord. White matter damage is responsible for the vast majority of subsequent functional loss.

Neural stem cells (NSCs) have been identified as the cells that help in the recovery of this type of injury. Therefore, transplantation of NSCs has the potential to harvest functional repair and recovery in the injury and diseases of the central nervous system, including spinal cord injury. These Neural stem cells, which are the precursors of neurons and glia cells, can be derived both from human embryonic stem cells (hESCs) and iPSC. (1, 2)

Oligodendrocytes are the central nervous system cells that surround and insulate the axons (the nerve fibers) through which a nerve's electrical messages are sent. Scientists, since 2005, have known that hESCs can make oligodendrocyte progenitors cells (OPC), which can improve the motor functions in rats with acute spinal cord injury. Induced pluripotent stem (iPS) cells have also demonstrated similar capability. (3) Demyelination is central to the pathology of the SCI, and its reversal by means of injecting oligodendrocyte progenitor cells would be revolutionary in this field.

In 2010, based on strong preclinical data from animal studies, and after a prolonged application process by Geron, the FDA finally approved the first embryonic stem cell treatment trial in humans for spinal cord injury. Proprietary oligodendrocyte progenitor cells called GRNOPC1, derived from embryonic stem cells, were used. The fifth and final patient in this Phase I trial was treated on 16 Nov. 2011 at the Stanford University School of Medicine. (4) Dr. Steinberg applied about 2 million of these cells directly into the injured area of the patient's spinal cord. The patients then entered an intensive rehabilitation program. All patients were reported to have responded well to this treatment and the implants. The trial was limited to patients who had been injured within 14 days and had only non-penetrating damage to a specific region of their thoracic spine.

This phase I Trial in patients with spinal cord injury earned a $25 million award from the California Institute for Regenerative Medicine (CIRM). Despite this funding, the trial stalled in late 2011, mostly due to financial concerns. At that point, under intense criticism, Geron withdrew from this field entirely, citing strategic business reasons. In early 2013, Geron's hESC-related assets, including the FDA-approved clinical trial, were bought by BioTime Inc. In 2014, Asterias Biotherapeutics, a subsidiary of BioTime Inc., was awarded $14.3 million by the California Institute for Regenerative Medicine (CIRM), to begin a new FDA-approved Phase I-IIa clinical trial. Asterias will use the same OPC1cells in 13 new patients with sub-acute, complete cervical spinal cord injury. Patient enrolment is expected in 2015.

Unlike in 2010, when Geron was the first and only player in the field, Asterias now faces tough competition. StemCells, a biotechnology company in California, has already treated 12 patients in a safety study with a different type of stem cell. More advanced trials are now expected to test the effectiveness of these cells. Another biotechnology company, Neuralstem of Maryland, also received regulatory approval in January 2013, to begin human tests of its stem cell product that is progressing well. With progress in iPSC technology, their potential to provide plentiful autologous cells for clinical use is also helping the field. Studies are showing a promise of inducing cellular plasticity in patients suffering from chronic cervical SCI. (5)

Leaving pluripotent ES cells and iPS cells behind, scientists are forging ahead with another line of research based on the knowledge that olfactory (smell sensing) nerve cells in the nose can regenerate freely. Studies on laboratory animals have shown that olfactory cells are helpful in regeneration of nerve cells elsewhere in the body. Based on these findings, a UK and Polish team recently performed a transplant procedure on a few spinal cord injury patients, using the patients' own olfactory nerve cells, with remarkable results. One of these patients, previously wheelchair-bound, is now able to walk with a walker, making international news headlines.

In scientific circles, however, these case reports are not taken as proof of efficacy, and randomized, controlled, double blind trials need to be performed before the true nature of benefits from these procedures can gain recognition as a treatment. This is to prove that a new therapy will work consistently, and not only in a single, random patient. In the mean time, anyone suffering from a recent spinal cord injury should look for stem cell trials enrolling new patients.

Despite promising, pre-clinical data, animal studies showing functional improvement and anecdotal case reports like the one above, there still are no definitive answers for patients suffering from a spinal cord injury. A variety of cellular therapies are being tested in novel clinical trials including OPCs, fetal-derived NSCs, and Schwann cells, but the final outcomes are pending. (6) Hope however is strong and the progress is being made, though results cannot come fast enough for more than 3 million people.

# Chapter 21

# STEM CELL AND HIV DISEASE

*"There are only two ways to live your life.*
*One is as though nothing is a miracle.*
*The other is as though everything is a miracle."*
*~Albert Einstein*

**The Berlin Patient**

In the ancient world, supernatural events better known as "miracles" were so common that before I can run down the list, you will run out of patience. In Pagan life-style miracles were everyday events. Great public institutions were built around them and their influence can be seen in every religious belief since then. For the ancients, miracles were just how the world worked. Gods had lots of power whereas common people had none. The big gap was filled by prophets and magicians who had the power to intercede, and people could get extra power by listening to, and following the prophets. In the modern world, miracles are exceptional; they need explanation. We have scientific facts and laws of thermodynamics, of motion, of energy, of gravity, etc. to explain how the world works. The ancients didn't know these laws so they didn't have to follow them.

In every age, all that was not understood or was unexplained was handed to the divine as its realm, but we now know things happen on account of the laws of nature. Things fall according to the laws of gravity, a fire burns because of the laws of chemistry, the sun, the moon and the stars cross the sky in accordance with the laws of physics, and a dice lands according to the laws of probability.

The more knowledge of laws of nature we have, the more likely we are to have a rational or scientific explanation for such miracles. For those who have a good understanding of how the world works based on the known laws, they will be certain that a law of nature is behind the perceived miracles even when they are not entirely sure what that law of nature may be. Because we are sure there are laws of nature at work, and that things happen in accordance with these laws, we understand that everything that happens—has a mechanical and impersonal cause.

The most often attested business of miracles was and still is health; and by far the greatest number of shrines and deities are busy answering such prayers. A large number of gods are essentially hailed as healers. Even in modern history there are often reported healing miracles. Here is the story of one such miracle.

*"What you seek is seeking you."*
*~Rumi*

"Berliner of the year" -2008, as reported in the German newspaper *Berliner Morgenpost*, was not a German, rather an American male, born in Seattle, WA, who can be described as living an adventurous life, traveling, studying, and exploring his sexuality in the 90s when he contracted HIV. Testing HIV positive for a young gay male was not an uncommon event in those days. Just like other HIV patients, he underwent treatment with AZT, followed by standard retroviral medications.

At the time of his diagnosis, he was traveling and working in Europe eventually deciding to live in Berlin, Germany. He later developed leukemia, a common but serious complication that many patients encounter at some point during their HIV positive life. Oncologist Dr. Gero Huetter, at Charité Hospital in Berlin, treated his patient's leukemia with chemotherapy which failed and the next standard procedure was a bone marrow transplant. On 6th of February 2007, after a total body irradiation which kills the patient's own blood forming cells, a matched donor was selected and bone marrow transplant was performed. The first attempt was not successful and patient underwent a second transplant. This time the stem cells from the donor's marrow reconstituted the blood and blood cells in the patient and on additional testing he was cured of leukemia.

The treatment also had a very pleasant side effect; it got rid of the HIV virus. (7)

Yes! The patient was cured of HIV, the first person in the history of HIV and AIDS who tested negative, after being HIV positive for a number of years. Since the transplant, he has undergone repeated tests, having almost every tissue of his body from his brain to his rectum biopsied. All tests have been negative. The patient no longer has HIV. The viral antibody levels kept dropping and the virus has remained undetectable. T-cell level (CD4 count) continued to increase, reaching that of a person who never had HIV. He no longer requires medications and has told reporters that he has had unprotected anal intercourse with HIV-positive men since his treatment but has himself remained negative, which means he is now immune to HIV. This is someone who had 2 serious illnesses before the stem cell treatment and only a slim chance of survival at best, and who is now living disease-free.

A miracle? Many claimed exactly that. Though I am not sure how people like Pat Robertson will explain this miracle of God that helped this openly gay man rid of HIV while innocent babies born in God-fearing, church-going families remain HIV positive. Sorry! I digress.

Media from around the world descended on Berlin to report on this major development. The patient, still weak and recovering from a major ordeal, was not ready to be bombarded by this media circus and chose to remain anonymous at that time. Instead he was referred in reports and news as the "Berlin Patient". His real name, later revealed, is Timothy Ray Brown, who bears the cross to be the only human who has ever been cured of HIV, not by a miracle, but by an innovative use of stem cells.

Here is how this "miracle" transpired. Viruses have the innate ability to infect cells. Once they get inside the cell they inject their nuclear material into the cell's nucleus and take control of the cell, hijacking its protein generation machinery. This helps replicate the virus and infect more and more cells. Each virus has its own way of doing this. The HIV virus uses a peculiar way of entry into the human T cells. It engages the host receptor, CCR5 (less frequently CXCR4), to gain entry. Therefore, if a person's T-lymphocytes do not have this CCR5 receptor, the HIV virus cannot enter the cells. It so happens that due to a rare genetic defect (delta 32) less than 1% of humans do not have CCR5 receptors and therefore no entry for the virus. A delta 32 mutation in their genes practically closes the door on HIV. (8)

We all get two copies of every gene, one from each parent. If both copies of the gene in a person have this delta 32 mutation, the cells will not have an entry receptor and would therefore be immune to HIV. Though it is rare for someone to have delta 32 mutations on both copies, oncologist Dr. Gero Huetter, was able to find a matching donor for Timothy. This donor had just the recipe for cure; a good tissue match for the leukemia and 2 copies of the delta 32 mutation. Timothy Brown was transplanted with the marrow stem cell from this donor; after Timothy's own cells were destroyed by radiation, the newly transplanted blood cells demonstrated complete immunity to the virus. The remaining viruses in the tissues were not able to infect these donor cells and the HIV virus was slowly killed by the new healthy immune cells. These HIV-immune donor cells could resist the virus but the virus could not resist them. The battle was finally won but unfortunately only for one. Several attempts to repeat this procedure have failed with patients dying from their primary disease.

Other researchers have attempted bone marrow transplants, without the delta 32 mutations, for HIV positive patients in the hope of a cure, however without success. Two such patients were treated in Boston, both showed absence of the virus for a few weeks after treatment, but the HIV virus became detectable in one patient after 12 weeks and the other after 32 weeks of ceasing antiretroviral therapy. It remains that Timothy Brown, "The Berlin Patient," is still the only one who has ever been completely cured of his HIV infection after a stem cell transplant. In June of 2013, Timothy told the Seattle Times, "I don't want to be the only person cured of HIV".

# Chapter 22

# DISEASE IN A DISH

**The Role of Stem Cells in Drug Discovery and Drug Delivery**

After learning all the basic sciences and the neat tricks that take place in laboratories, you are now well-equipped to understand the finer details of stem cell applications in drug discovery, drug delivery and therapeutic interventions.

Traditionally, medicinal products were substances found in nature. All ancient medical practices used plant and animal products and minerals to prepare their therapeutic concoctions. Flowers, leaves, roots and barks of trees, dried testicular extracts of bulls, dried placenta, horn of rhinoceros and powdered ivory, pearl, gold and silver were all part of this armamentarium, discovered not by scientific methods, but by trial and error, and knowledge spread by the word of mouth.

Ancient Sumerians used willow; a salicylate-rich plant and the source of modern aspirin for treatment of pain. Digitalis was used by the ancient Romans for heart failure. South American natives discovered cinchona bark, as a source of quinine and used it as an effective treatment for malaria. Even today, new plant-based molecules are constantly being tested by pharmaceutical companies for possible beneficial effects. Over time, the mode of drug discovery however moved away from trial and error and generational experience.

In 1856, alchemy took a new turn. A professor of chemistry, August Hofmann, gave one of his bright 18 year old students, William Perkins, a challenge to synthesize quinine. His very first attempt failed to create quinine but serendipity was watching over him. He noticed a purple portion in the solution. This aniline compound turned out to be a suitable dye for creating beautiful silk and other textiles. Instead of synthesizing quinine, Perkin patented the dye and started his own business, mass producing it. Production of other synthetic aniline dyes followed; since aniline was noted to have analgesic effects it started the revolution of using synthetic substances for medicinal use. In the late 19th century, while trying to modify synthetic dyes to treat African sleeping sickness, Paul Ehrlich discovered the first organic arsenical drug, Salvarsan, which was later used as a treatment for syphilis. (1)

In 1932, Bayer started exploring medical applications of other synthetic dyes, and came up with sulfonamide drugs as antimicrobial agents. In the following years, penicillin was developed into a synthetic antibiotic. Both these drugs were highly popular in the 1940s due to the demand in the World War II and the post war era. Until then much of the U.S. pharmacopoeia was composed of drugs of herbal origin.

As time passed, new developments in the synthetic medicine industry, allowed for extraction, purification, and standardization of natural molecules. Plant and animal-derived substances were made measurable, reproducible and testable. After formal testing, experimentation and patient research, many of these ancient remedies at therapeutic doses were found either ineffective or with serious side effects. Still, several of the traditional plant remedies are in use today, though in their refined forms, such as Aspirin, Atropine, Capsaicin, Cocaine, Colchicine, Digoxin, Ephedrine, Ergotamine, Metformin, Opium, Quinidine, Scopolamine, to name a few.

The new drug development process involves understanding of the steps in the pathological development of a disease. Identification of a step that can be influenced, then leads to the discovery of a substance that can impact the disease limiting step. An example would be anti-inflammatory, pain medications like Ibuprofen or Naprosyn.

As a result of diseases or injury there is tissue inflammation, and the chemical substances that promote this inflammation cause pain. The mechanisms through which these inflammatory substances are produced have enzymatic steps. One of the key steps in this pathway involves the cyclooxygenase enzyme. Once this was identified, chemical molecules were developed to block cyclooxygenase enzyme thus limiting inflammation and reducing pain. That is how all the different anti-inflammatory drugs work, and we call it the "mechanism of action" of that drug.

CLINICAL TRIALS:

Scientists and researchers, in the early stages of drug discovery, try to understand the disease and discover the right molecule to interact with the right target. The problem with this model of development of synthetic substances is that no one knows how they will act inside the human body and whether they are safe. In order to answer these questions we need to establish safety and efficacy which requires animal testing. This is accomplished by breeding mice, rabbits, or other appropriate animal models that are genetically or physically modified to produce the relevant symptoms. These animals are then treated with the drug to see if the symptoms get better: **Pre-clinical Trial.**

Even if both, efficacy and safety, in animal models is confirmed there is no telling how humans will respond to the drug. The next step is to try the medicine on a few healthy volunteers, (10s of patients) to test for safety at different dose levels: **Phase I Trial.**

If the drug appears safe it moves to the next step of assessment. Patients suffering from the disease are tested for effectiveness. This is conducted in a larger group (100s of subjects). These trials are designed to assess how well the drug works: **Phase II Trials.**

Only a small number of clinical trials move past Phase II; either because the drug is not effective or is too toxic. The next phase is randomized, controlled and multicenter trials involving large patient groups (1000s of patients). These are the most expensive, time-consuming and difficult trials: **Phase III trials.**

The discovery and development of new medicines is, therefore, a long and expensive process. Taking a drug from early understanding of the disease and identification of an appropriate drug molecule to its clinical testing, and finally to market, generally takes more than a decade and costs anywhere from a few million to over a billion dollars. Unfortunately only one out of ten successfully identified drug molecules make it to the market.

**Designer Stem Cells.**

Despite the vision that an average person has of stem cell medicine which involves stem cells being injected in the body where they replace the damaged or diseased cell, in reality it is only a small part of the story and only one of the several mechanisms by which stem cells work in clinical medicine. Studies have shown that the direct conversion of stem cells to local tissue cells is responsible for only a limited range of the benefits that stem cells provide in recovery. The more likely mechanisms are the release of substances from stem cells into local tissue that cause immune modulation, decrease inflammation, growth factor production, and stimulation of the local tissue stem cells.

One completely unrelated application and benefit is their use in drug development and testing. Acquiring human cells is not easy; no one is willing to part with their liver, brain or heart tissue. Human cells are, therefore, not readily available in quantities needed to perform drug testing. Embryonic stem cells can certainly change this predicament. However, embryonic stem cells can be even harder to acquire. The introduction of iPS cells has changed this paradigm. It is now easy to take cells from a patient with a particular disease and program them to become pluripotent (more stem-like). These cells can then be coaxed into a specific cell type, for example, a cell type that is diseased. An example would be nudging pluripotent cells down a biological pathway to form motor neurons in a model of ALS (Lou Gehrig's disease). In this manner the development of a disease and the candidates for its treatment can be studied.

Stem cell models offer new opportunities to improve the method in which pharmaceutical companies identify lead candidates for new drugs, and expedite their reach to the market. This model also allows testing for any toxic effects on heart or liver cells; two common toxicities that limit the use of most drugs. Pharmaceutical companies now routinely use iPSC-derived cardiomyocytes (heart cells) and hepatocytes (liver cells) as high-throughput models to assess toxicity for drugs in development. (3)

Currently available models fail to fully recapitulate the complexity of the genetic and environmental impact on disease onset and progression, especially in progressive neurodegenerative diseases such as Parkinson's, Alzheimer's or

ALS. Diseases of the brain are particularly hard to study because extracting neurons from a living patient is difficult and risky. On the other hand, post-mortem assessment only shows the final stages of the disease. Current animal models are not optimal for the crucial drug-development stage of research. In these situations, induced Pluripotent Stem Cells (iPSCs) offer opportunities for proof-of-concept studies and a platform for drug discovery research.

iPSCs technology is providing innovative tools for drug development and toxicity screening, using patient-derived iPSCs. Additionally, these cells can be generated from patients, irrespective of the familial or sporadic nature of a disease. Regenerative medicine techniques are now able to generate functioning mini livers, mini kidneys and clusters of heart cells, which can be effective substitutes for toxicity testing during preclinical trials. This will allow analysis of certain aspects of drug metabolism and probable side effects. These "disease in a dish" models are now available for Parkinson's, Alzheimer's, ALS, Huntington's and many other ailments, providing valuable insights and an enhanced promise for cure. (4) Today, the use of iPS cells in the pharmaceutical industry is becoming routine practice for a variety of disease models for rare and common diseases alike. (5, 6)

Research in this area is moving at a fast pace...

In 2006, Shinya Yamanka reprogrammed mice cells into a stem-like state.

In 2007, the same trick was demonstrated in humans.

In 2008, iPSCs-derived neuronal cells were developed from an ALS patient.

In 2010, a Stanford group converted skin cells into neurons by direct reprogramming.

Preclinical studies are advancing everyday towards new and promising ideas. How diseases can be studied is opening up new doors to treatment options with iPS technology at the heart of this advancement. Scientists have used iPS-derived nerve cells to study a range of neurological disorders, including

Alzheimer's, Parkinson's, and Huntington's disease, which are also being used as models for testing potential treatments. (7,8,9,10)

In other areas, iPS-based cells have been developed for a range of diseases, for example, blindness from age-related macular degeneration, (11) spinal cord injuries, (12) and osteoporosis and cartilage damage. (13) iPS cell technology has also offered an entirely new platform for understanding the causes of diseases of the heart, (16, 17) kidney, (18) liver, (19) and pancreas. (20)

Researchers have developed insulin-producing cells derived from iPS cells, which are being tested in mice with positive results. This technology also offers tools to evaluate potential drugs for the treatment of these diseases. In human studies, scientists have converted human skin cells into blood cells through direct reprogramming, altogether bypassing the iPS cell stage. A new frontier of cellular reprogramming for disease research has come on the horizon with this new approach. (21)

Stem cell–related technologies have exciting potential for improved disease models and innovative therapies. At the Bluefield project, researchers have directly reprogrammed fibroblasts into multipotent neural stem cells with a single factor. (22) Investigators at The J. David Gladstone Institute are using patient-derived, induced, pluripotent stem cells to study novel human cell-culture models of ALS , Alzheimer's, Parkinson's, and Huntington's disease. Researchers have now shown that interneuron precursors transplanted into brains of AD mouse models develop into functional interneurons, integrate into microcircuits, improve brain rhythms, and reduce cognitive dysfunction.

The highly pursued and pertinent questions in stem cell research are...

1 - What are the main regulators of stem cells?
2 - What role do genetics and epigenetics play in this regards?
3 - What factors influence stem cell renewal, differentiation and growth?
4 - What role does the environment, including the growth medium plays in influencing the critical characteristics of stem cells?
5 - How can the useful characteristics of stem cells that are coming to light be utilized for clinical benefits?

All these areas are making rapid gains, thanks to the advances in DNA sequencing technology, bioinformatics and computational biology. Significant progress has been made in directing embryonic, adult and induced stem cells to differentiate along specific lineages in vitro. *(23)*

The future is looking more and more promising with each new model of a disease developing in a dish and then moving on to possible solutions for complex medical problems that have plagued humans for millennia.

# Chapter 23

# STEM CELLS AND AGING

*Life would be infinitely happier if we could only be born at the age of 80 and gradually approach 18. ~ Mark Twain*

## Tithonus and the Elixir of Life

Search of immortality and eternal youth is as old as the history of medicine itself. Though so far this search has failed, it has given birth to myths and tales such as "elixir of life" and "fountain of youth". Old age and death are fears we all live with. For eons, we have dreamed of overcoming aging and death but never have we got close to an answer. Therefore, eternal youth and immortality became a frequently sought-after gift in legends. Failing to find real and practical means, people sought magical ways to restore their youth.

In Greek mythology, gods and goddesses were considered eternal. In many ancient mythologies, they gained eternal youth and achieved agelessness by eating ambrosia. Many blur the difference between agelessness and youth which are two entirely different attributes. When goddess Eos fell in love with Tithonus, a mortal Titan from Troy, she begged Zeus to bestow immorality on her human lover. However, she overlooked to ask for eternal youth and therefore Tithonus got old, decrepit and miserable, forever begging to die while she lost all interest in him.

The average human on the other hand, unable to achieve god-like characteristics, settled for stories and myths. The stories of these myths have been appearing forever in writings such as Herodotus, Alexander romance, and biographies of explorers like Juan Ponce de León of Spain. Stories of elixir of life have also been noted in the tales of indigenous people of South America and the Caribbean, who spoke of the mythical land of Bimini, where there existed the springs with magical restorative powers in its water. (1)

Just like Alexander, who was said to have been searching for the river of youth in Asia, Juan Ponce de León was allegedly looking for it in Florida. (1) Today in St. Augustine, Florida (the oldest city in the U.S.) there exists a fountain frequented by tourists. Unfortunately, the elderly visitors who drink from this sulfur spring do not turn into teenagers.

In the Buddhist sect of Tibet there is the belief of a place called Shambhala, a mystical and sacred place near Mongolia or Tibet, which also possesses the springs of such waters that give eternal life. Travelers' accounts and historians have both mentioned the longevity and youthfulness of these people. Hindu sacred texts mention immortals that are believed to be alive throughout the universal existence. There are accounts of yogis and swamis who have witnessed these immortal beings and have themselves conquered old age and death. These yogis are claimed to dwell in the mountain ranges of the Himalayas bordering Nepal and Tibet.

In ancient China, various emperors also sought this fabled elixir. The ancient Chinese believed that ingesting long-lasting precious substances such as jade, gold or hematite conferred the same longevity on the person who consumed them. They developed the idea of drinkable gold in the 3$^{rd}$ century BC. The most famous Chinese alchemical books describe in detail the creation of elixirs for immortality that contain mercury, sulfur, and arsenic, all of them ironically are poisonous.

In the Arab culture is the myth of Aab-i-Hayat, supposedly found in paradise, and has the same properties as that of elixir of life in Greek tradition. In ancient Persian texts, the Cup of Jamshid is described as a cup of divination, long possessed by the rulers of ancient Iran. The cup, filled with an elixir of immortality was said to reveal deep truths, and the whole world was reflected in it.

Despite all the myths and claims, technically-speaking, neither immortality nor eternal youth is scientifically feasible. Immortal means incapable of dying, and eternal means guaranteed existence for eternity. Well! Immortality is not possible in science because even if we overcome all diseases, cure all ailments, and find effective treatment for aging, the possibility of accidental death or ability to take one's own life still remains. On the other hand, the principle of entropy (the concept of inevitable disorder and degeneration of everything) prevents eternal anything. Based on the principle of entropy, everything is under decay, no matter how slow the rate.

You may call it semantics, but the term "indefinite lifespan", represents a more achievable state than immortality, since it implies freedom from death by aging or infirmity but does not make one unable to die. Since protection from aging does not guarantee survival, there is hope to achieve something like that. But even an indefinite life span is not optimal if you forget to ask for "negligible senescence" (a more feasible alternative for eternal youth).

Now that I have negotiated you down from "immortality" to "indefinite lifespan" and "eternal youth" to "negligible senescence", let's clarify something. These are not politically correct terms like "vertically challenged" for short or "metabolically challenged" for fat. These are actual scientific concepts around which heated debates and annual conferences are being held. So please take it seriously.

The key figure behind the concept of *Strategies for Engineered Negligible Senescence* (SENS) is the British bio-gerontologist, Aubrey de Grey. The term "negligible senescence" was first used to describe organisms like hydra which do not show signs of aging. The next term, "engineered negligible senescence", was coined by Aubrey de Grey in his Mitochondrial Free Radical Theory of Aging. The word "strategy" was added later, to complete the term as a proposed model for steps to overcome aging or senescence. This is a goal-directed approach to the science of aging. It is controversial, with no shortage of critics, but that's not the subject for this book. The point is, just like the ancients, even in today's science there is a concerted effort to stop or slow down aging and it is not all about cosmetic change. Most of the degenerative diseases are essentially diseases of aging or they are the result of aging processes of the nucleus, the mitochondria, the vessels, the heart, the pancreas, the kidney, you name it. This search for agelessness is based on many concepts and theories. Some of the more accepted theories of aging are discussed below.

## Cell Suicide

When adult body cells divide, the small protective cover at the end of their chromosomes, called "telomere", is shortened a bit with each division and eventually runs out its entire length. At this point the cell stops to divide, a stage called replicative senescence. Normal cells, therefore, have a finite lifespan. In other words, all cells are programmed to die. This programmed cell death (apoptosis) also occurs in response to DNA damage. (2) It is essentially a protective mechanism to prevent division of old, senile, or abnormal cells, which may have damaged DNA or other functional abnormalities. (3)

Apoptosis is often referred to as "cell suicide", since the cell itself manufactures the killer protein P53. When cells grow too large, or too fast, a tumor suppressor gene calls for P53, which triggers cell suicide or "Apoptosis". Apoptosis is characterised by changes within the cell, including nuclear condensation, and cytoplasmic shrinkage. (4) The cell then produces proteolytic enzymes that destroy the cell.

Cells appear to have a memory of how many times they have divided and even if frozen and later thawed they seem to remember the population-doubling level at which they were preserved. (5) That means cells are preprogrammed for a fixed number of cell cycles and no more.

## Programmed Senescence:

In the state before the cells die and after the replicative senescence, cells can no longer divide but change into a rather flat shape, secreting substances that cause inflammation and degenerative changes related to aging. These cells stay metabolically active and resist apoptosis or cell death to some extent, but the programmed intrinsic mechanism tries to kill them anyway. If this mechanism is disrupted for any reason, the senescent cells continue to live their senile existence with their short telomeres. These senile cells cause a lot of damage by producing chemical signals that incite inflammation leading to cancer, heart disease, and dementia.

**Telomerase Theory of Aging:**

Telomeres are tandem repeats of DNA. They are necessary for the maintenance of proper chromosomal structure. Functionally, they appear to serve like the cap of a shoelace and protect the chromosomes from degradation or fraying. Our body does know how to make the telomeres long again; there is an enzyme, called telomerase, which can recover the lost telomere length. However, except for the stem cells (and cancer cells), the gene responsible for this enzyme is silenced and sealed after birth in all adult cells. We have not yet figured out how to reactivate this gene.

The problem is that you cannot ingest or even inject telomerase; it is only effective inside the cell nucleus. All cells intrinsically know how to make their own telomerase, we just need to find and remind them the way to signal its production. In recent years some commercial products and medications have claimed the ability to increase telomerase in cells. However, peer-reviewed scientific proof of their efficacy is still missing. Some Chinese herbal extracts have been found to stimulate expression of telomerase. Silymarin, from milk thistle, and astragalus also make the same claim.

Short telomeres are associated with a rise in mortality, independent of age. This has been proven in patients suffering from Progeria, a rare genetic disorder. Patients with Progeria are characterized by premature aging. These kids are born with short telomeres. They age rapidly and die very early looking many times older than their chronological age.

It is possible that the telomere length is the body's clock, which tells it how old it really is, and simply lengthening telomeres can possibly reset this clock. Researchers have experimented with mice (mice normally have long telomerase) by genetically blocking their telomerase. This resulted in terrible degeneration of their bodies. In the next step, telomerase was turned back on to see if the mice become young again and the results were astonishing. The mice regrew their atrophied tissue, they got smarter and stronger and their hair grew back when telomerase was turned on.

Organisms that have either ample telomerase like hydra, or a large number of stem cells like planarian, can replicate and regenerate without senescence or apoptosis. In lab experiments, the addition of telomerase to cell cultures increases the length of telomeres in these cells and the cells continue to divide, and not only exceed the maximal life-span of the normal cells, they divide at the rate of younger cells. (6) Thus, telomerase is capable of extending cellular longevity. (7) However, besides suppressing cellular senescence, this perpetual replication and potential immortality may also promote tumor formation.

## Free Radical Theory of Aging

Normal metabolism in all cells leads to the production of by-products that are damaging to cells. The most physiologically significant are the reactive oxygen species (ROS). An example is superoxide, produced in the mitochondria. If there are no protective antioxidants present, the superoxide can cause damage to important biomolecules including DNA, (8) and if the damage is too great, the cell undergoes apoptosis, resulting in a shorter lifespan. Evidence of this is seen in patients with Down syndrome, who have a shortened lifespan due to the presence of a high amount of oxidative stress. (9)

Studies show that an increased level of oxygen radicals is inversely proportionate to the lifespan of organisms. (10) It is interesting to note that the molecule most essential for life, oxygen, can also be responsible for most of our destruction. Fortunately, cells do know how to defend themselves from the damaging effects of oxidative stress, with the help of antioxidants, such as, vitamin C, vitamin E, $\beta$-carotene and enzymes like superoxide dismutase (SOD) and glutathione peroxidase. (11)

## Stem Cell Theory of Aging:

Aging stem cells play a critical role in determining the effects of aging on organ function and ultimately on the lifespan. Aging has both quantitative and qualitative effects on stem cells, including self-renewal, response to signals and decreased functioning. The number and activity of stem cells has been correlated with the progression of aging. This is the newest approach to intercept aging and holds a lot of promise. Which of these theories are closest to the truth and which will deliver the real fountain of youth, remains to be seen.

**Anti-Aging Approaches:**

A diverse range of regenerative medicine approaches and therapies are either under investigation or in development. The ultimate goal, whether stated or implied, is the achievement of a state of negligible senescence. Much research is also being conducted in the sciences of genetics, which, if successful, is expected to allow manipulation of the aging process; no wonder the topic of aging and anti-aging is so often in the media.

Candidate approaches to prevention of aging include:

**Genetic Fountain of Youth:**

At the genetic level, techniques that can turn on the telomerase gene, allowing cells to have an unlimited amount of divisions without the telomere shortening and risk to DNA integrity, is another possible way to maintain youth. Researchers have found that when they injected the "longevity gene" into aging mice, they stepped up the production of new adult stem cells, thus fending off the decline that would have been expected from normal aging. Similar research is underway for humans.

**Molecular Fountain of Youth:**

Natural molecules like sirtuins (proteins known to regulate aging) which are thought to play a role in lifespan extension in mammals have been found in high concentration in the hematopoietic stem cells (HSCs), they are believed to improve the regenerative capacity of these stam cells. Scientific studies are now providing evidence that aging-associated degeneration can be reversed by a number of these sirtuins. (12)

**Cellular Fountain of Youth**

And then we have our own tissue-specific stem cells which persist throughout our lifespan to repair and maintain our tissues, but as we age, their self-renewal and differentiation potential becomes diminished or deregulated, so scientists are looking at ways to improve or enhance this function in an attempt to impede the age-related degeneration of tissues. Another mechanism could be to externally supplement our bodies with stem cells.

**Herbal Fountain of Youth:**

Some herbal supplements are known to stimulate the release of natural stem cells, for example, Fuciodens in brown algae, (13) or blue green algae (one of the most primitive life forms on earth) containing AFA (Aphanizomenon flos-aquae). These organisims have both plant and animal features but they act more like primitive bacteria. Edible blue-green algae includes a large variety, the most common ones known for their health benefits are Spirulina and Aphanizomenon flos-aquae, both of which have been used as food for centuries. More recently, their use has been associated with stem cell health, cell mobilization and positive immune-modulatory effects. Some species of blue green algae have also been reported to have cholesterol-lowering, anti-cancer and glucose-reduction activity. (14)

**Hormonal Fountain of Youth:**

In order to ensure survival of the race, the human body is programmed to produce and release hormones and chemicals to help restore and maintain health during the reproductive years. However, as we go past the reproductive peak, the need, and thus the levels of these hormones such as sex hormones, growth hormones and melatonin, decline. Traditional medicine assumes that "as we age our hormone levels go down", but the new paradigm states, "we age because our hormone levels go down". Therefore, replacing and maintaining these hormones in a youthful range can maintain youth for a longer period of time. This, however, is a complex cacophony which needs very skilled, fine tuning by a physician who is well-trained in hormone optimization to turn it into a symphony again.

**Pharmaceutical Fountain of Youth:**

A natural drug in the soil of Easter Island - rapamycin – (the "forever young" drug), (15) discovered in the shadows of the island's famous statues, is touted to prevent the signs of aging in the brain and is being tested for treatment of Alzheimer's disease and Progeria Syndrome that causes children to age at a greatly exaggerated rate.

**Physical Fountain of Youth:**

The benefits described above for the herbal supplements, dietary choices, anti-aging medicines, plus the benefits of stem cells are all combined in one easy recipe; physical activity. Regular moderate exercise is known and proven to maintain healthy and young heart, lungs, and blood vessels. Increases in stem cell concentration, improved blood flow as well as increased metabolism have all been associated with regular exercise. Exercise also releases health and youth-enhancing hormones and brain chemicals that promote wellbeing.

# Chapter 24

# HEALTHY STEM CELLS LIFESTYLE

*Healing is a matter of time, but it is also a matter of opportunity.*
*~Hippocrates (460 BC - 370 BC)*

Performing an autopsy is not the most pleasant experience. The first time I attended an autopsy, I was a medical student. I stood around the cold steel table along with another 20 some students, a few residents and the medical examiner running a commentary while cutting open the chest and abdominal cavities.

The air in the room was warm and stuffy. Even though it was silent, you could sense the presence of a lot of keen observers around you even with your eyes closed. There was the peculiar dead body smell, hallmark of a hospital morgue. As the abdominal cavity opened the smell in the room went from unpleasant to nauseating; everyone covered their noses in a futile attempt. The middle-aged male whose body lay nude and motionless on the table had remained unclaimed and unidentified and had started to decompose a little. Unlike CSI Miami or NCIS, this autopsy was not for the determination of a criminal intent or cause of death but a demonstration of postmortem skills to the students and trainees.

My imagination drifted for a few seconds wondering who this man was. The sound of an electrical tool quickly redirected my attention. The chest cavity was being cut open with a small electric saw, cracked wider with the help of retractors, so that everyone can peek in. Very few brave souls attempted to get any closer than they already were.

The medical examiner pointed out the heart, liver, stomach, pancreas, major arteries and veins, etc. and then he directed our attention to two pieces of black charcoal-like substance on either side of the heart. They didn't look like human tissue. Had I not seen the chest opened right in front of my eyes, I would have thought they came from outside the body.

The question the examiner put to us was, "What is this?" No one answered. My brain started working at a quantum speed, I noticed that they sat where the lungs should be but I knew what the human lungs looked like; I had seen pictures in text books, seen pristine specimens preserved in the anatomy lab and seen live lungs during surgeries. This was not lung tissue; then what? Someone said, "a foreign body". I smiled at the responder's foolishness; how can such a large foreign body get in there? Before I could complete my thought, the medical examiner said, "Well! In a way it is." I looked at him with great surprise. He smiled and said these are lungs, but most of this tissue is smoke and cigarette substrate from outside and part of it is cancer tissue from smoking. My jaw dropped. That's what a smoker's lung looks like? Not the pink, spongy, glistening, air inflated tissue but a rather solid-looking, leathery-appearing, dark, shrunken, irregular, dark and ugly figure. If the harm smoking does to the inside of the body was visible on the outside, no one would ever smoke; I thought to myself, reaffirming not to ever smoke.

I completed the autopsy, washed up and went across the street with some friends to grab a bite. Standing right outside the restaurant was the medical examiner who just taught us the autopsy. Talking to some people, he tossed the butt of a cigarette he just finished and lit up another one. By the time we got near him he was almost half done with the second one as well. I must have been staring at him pretty hard, because as I passed close to him he looked straight at me and asked, "What"? I was startled, as if I woke up from sleep. I said, "Nothing Sir" and moved my gaze, picked up my pace and rushed into the restaurant. My friend asked, "What's wrong?"

"Nothing", I said, and then I asked him how can this guy smoke after seeing the lungs of that dead smoker? My friend laughed and, as always, said "You think too much". That was the end of our discussion. Hunger took over, menu became a priority and the smell of BBQ made me forget everything else.

But I still think and wonder when I see a patient who is recovering from throat cancer caused by cigarettes, sitting outside the hospital smoking from the hole in his neck that now replaces his voice box. I think when I see a patient in the waiting room eating a beef burger and French fries, who has come back for his follow up visit after a heart bypass surgery, because his arteries were clogged with cholesterol, I think…….., when I see the man with several new tattoos and recall he was last in the hospital for treatment of hepatitis he got from a tattoo parlor…….When I see the woman standing under the sun exposing her shoulders in order to tan, and I can see the site we took a skin biopsy from to rule out skin cancer……. I think when I see the teenager speed by on his motorcycle without a helmet………. I think when I see the alcoholic, liver failure patient being brought into the hospital by his wife, with a beer can in his hand.

I still wonder, why do these people not think what they are doing to their bodies? I think if they don't take care of their body, which vessel are they going to live in? I wonder if they knew that their body has a natural healing system would they protect it or would they continue to do injurious things to it.

They say "From the bitterness of disease man learns the sweetness of health" but is not it too late to learn. May be my friends are right; I do think too much.

*"You were born with wings, why prefer to crawl through life?"*
*~ Rumi*

Ancient cultures understood the value of prevention, and depending on their philosophy of disease and cures, recommended modes of prevention of illness. Ancient Greeks encouraged the balancing of four fluids or 'humors' in the body; they advised a good balance with appropriate fluid intake, bloodletting and adjusting the frequency of sexual intercourse. Ancient Chinese advised a balance of vital energy or *qi* in the body, and the Indian system of Ayurveda medicine based its advice for preserving health in herbs, diet and physical treatments. Roman surgeons used tools that were boiled in hot water before each use. Acid and vinegar was used to wash wounds, all in an effort to prevent disease.

*Treatment without prevention is simply unsustainable.*
*~ Bill Gates*

In more recent years, the recommendations from physicians and philosophers have been to follow systematic measures, such as exercise or diet, and the maintenance of good hygiene in order to remain healthy. The concept of prevention of disease has continued to evolve along with our enlightenment regarding disease and prevention. With the spread of sexually-transmitted diseases like hepatitis and HIV, a more recent addition to the list of preventative measures has been the practice of 'safe sex'.

Prevention in the old paradigm was more focused on avoiding contact with infective agents, and limiting diet that would predispose to diseases like diabetes and high blood pressure. In the new paradigm, maintenance of health and prevention of diseases adds a new chapter of recommendations targeted towards keeping a healthy and robust system of repair and renewal in the body. This entails maintaining a high activity and number of stem cells in the body.

Research has repeatedly shown a direct correlation between the number of circulating stem cells and recovery from injury or disease. When two groups of stroke survivors were compared, based on the circulating stem cell count in their blood at the time of the stroke, the one that had a higher number of circulating stem cells had a more profound neurological recovery, as compared to the patient who had a lower stem cell count, (1,33)

Another study in heart disease patients showed a strong correlation between the number of circulating Endothelial Progenitor Cells (EPCs) (a type of circulating stem cell) and the risk for cardiovascular disease. The number of EPCs was found to be a better predictor of vascular reactivity than the existence or nonexistence of traditional cardiac risk factors. (2) Other researchers looked at the stem cell response after an acute heart attack and found that the stem cells and endothelial progenitor cells significantly increased after a heart attack, reaching a peak at 7 days, indicating the normal response to injury and recovery in the heart. (3)

Based on the knowledge that higher numbers of circulating stem cells increase chances of recovery, Granulocyte Colony-Stimulating Factor (G-CSF), a drug that mobilizes stem cells, was given to half the patients following acute myocardial infarction (heart attack). The other half was used as a control. At five month follow up, patients who received G-CSF (and in turn had mobilization of stem cells) showed a substantially higher pumping ability (ejection fraction) of the heart than those treated by conventional methods, without G-CSF. (4) Augmentation of circulating stem and progenitor cells using G-CSF and similar drugs have shown promising preclinical and early clinical results for several degenerative conditions. However, the use of these agents is limited by cost and side effects that prevent chronic administration.

Heart diseases and strokes are not the only diseases that show this correlation with stem cells. Patients with Alzheimer's have also been noted with reduced levels of circulating stem cells when compared to healthy individuals. Lower levels of stem cells also correlate with the severity of the disease. (5) Similarly, decreased numbers of stem cells have been noted in other ailments such as Migraine (6) & erectile dysfunction. (7)

Based on the above studies and many others like these, it has been established that a higher number of stem cells in circulation is a marker of better health. Finding ways to increase the intrinsic number of stem cells in the blood would be a good way to enhance health and wellness. And that's what "Healthy Stem Cell Lifestyle" means. Identifying diets, activities and supplements that can help achieve this goal all constitute the Healthy Stem Cell Lifestyle. Practicing healthy habits in general, which keep the body fit, also indirectly helps in maintaining this lifestyle. Factors that can help achieve this goal include, losing unhealthy habits, improving diet, exercise, supplements and use of certain medications.

> *"To keep the body in good health is a duty...otherwise we shall not be able to keep our mind strong and clear." ~ Buddha*

SMOKING:

Everyone knows that smoking is injurious to health; there is specific scientific evidence of adverse impact on stem cells both from smoking and second hand smoke (8). Adverse effect of tobacco smoke on SC includes both direct influences on the cell components and their regulatory mechanisms, as well as changes in SC microenvironment known as a SC niche. Nicotine is known to delay bone growth by influencing the two-step bone healing process:

a- Stem cells become cartilage.
b- Cartilage matures into bone. (9)

When smokers and non-smokers were compared on the basis of stem cell count in their blood, it was discovered that the number of endothelial progenitor cells increased after the cessation of smoking and decreased to previous levels again after resumption of smoking. (12)

EXERCISE:

*"Now there are more overweight people in America than average-weight people. So over-weight people are now average. Which means you've met your New Year's resolution"* ~Jay Leno

I know most people are sick of hearing about the benefits of exercise. It has been preached so often in doctor's offices that if one forgets, the table lamp can repeat it for you. But just because it has been said too many times, does not make it less important, absolutely not! So stop covering your ears, move those hands and listen. Moderate, regular exercise not only improves heart and vascular health, reduces obesity, prevents diabetes, decreases cancer risk, improves brain neuro transmitters, and supports lung function; it also directly and indirectly promotes stem cell growth. It is shown to increase vascular endothelial growth factor (VEGF) which stimulates growth of new blood vessels improving supply of oxygen and nutrients. (13) Exercise also stimulates the release of the brain derived neurotropic factor (BDNF) which increases the activity and number of stem cells in the brain memory center (14), and stem cell renewal is associated with less depression due to an increase in serotonin levels. Exercise till you sweat so you can get rid of the toxins in your body.

*Be melting snow. Wash yourself of yourself."*
*~Rumi,*

DIET and FOOD:

All diet has to be metabolized in the body. The mitochondria in every cell use this nutrition to produce energy. During this energy generation process some by-products are also manufactured which are injurious to the cells. These are called reactive oxygen species (ROS). In order to neutralize these bad boys we need anti-oxidants. A good diet needs a balance and a variety of nutrients, from good, fresh, natural sources, plus vitamins, minerals and water. When it comes to a balanced diet and healthy food choices there are few simple rules:

Calorie restriction: Limit the total number of calories in your diet; there is no substitute for it. Reducing fats and simple sugars in food and adding high-fiber elements helps accomplish this goal.

Pick the least-refined ingredients: The more unrefined and closer to natural form, the better for health. Polished rice, refined sugar, white flour, concentrated juices, processed canned fruits and vegetables are all bad for health. Eat fresh, whole fruits, whole grains, fresh vegetables, brown sugar or use natural sweeteners like honey, dates, figs, apple sauce, raisins, etc. to satisfy your sweet tooth. They have vitamins, minerals and antioxidants with a healthy dose of fiber.

Pick your food by color: Include as many colors as you can in your diet and this will allow inclusion of a variety of products and a wide array of vitamins, minerals and natural supplements. Bell peppers, carrots, turnips, celery, broccoli, cauliflower, eggplant, mushrooms, onion, ginger, garlic, turmeric, lemon, lime, beans, or chick peas, in your salad, can do you a lot of good. Following this, a few hours later, try to snack on a fruit plate that is just as colorful. Raspberry, blueberry, kiwi, plum, apricot, orange, pear, apple, peach, melon, mango, guava, papaya, pineapple, mangosteen, and lychee, are all good, but, may be not too many bananas or grapes. Remember, in general, darker the shade of color, more the antioxidant content.

Use liquid fats: If a fat gets hard at room temprature it will get hard in your arteries. In general animal fats are bad, plant fats are good. So reach for olive oil, avocados, peanuts, walnuts, and almonds; not butter, lard or margarine.

SLEEP:

> *"The moon stays bright when it doesn't avoid the night."*
> *~ Rumi*

Besides its other health benefits, good sleep has also been associated with faster recovery from illness. Sleep deprivation is reported as a factor in reduced stem cell proliferation. (15) Bone marrow transplant patients who experience good sleep after surgery exhibit better recovery than those who have impaired sleep. Two mechanisms have been suggested as the cause of this effect - melatonin and growth hormone. Both these substances are released during sleep and have been noted for their youth-promoting effect while their decline has been implicated in aging.

Sleep quality, its duration and melatonin levels, all decline with age, from an average of about 90 pg/ml in a thirty year old, to sometimes below 30 pg/ml in a seventy year old. Associated with this decline are the decreased proliferation, renewal and activity of neuronal stem cells especially in the memory area of the brain (Hippocampus). (16) Age-related growth hormone decline is also a well-established scientific fact and is associated with impaired cognitive and memory functions in animals and humans. This is possibly the result of the decreased number of neurons and stem cells in the hippocampus. (17, 18)

Considering what we have learned above, wouldn't it make sense to figure out how to make our body produce, release and sustain more adult stem cells? Are'nt we likely to reap amazing benefits like longevity, youth, optimum health, and peak performance with this approach. We already know that body has stem cells and these cells can heal. These cells move from the marrow to the injured tissue on demand and they have amazing powers to promote local healing as well as the ability to contribute to tissue repair by transforming and replacing damaged cells and tissues. Many scientific studies have found that adult stem cells can become heart cells, (19, 20) liver cells, (21, 22) pancreatic cells, (23, 24), muscle cells, (25, 26) lung cells, (27) cartilage, (28, 29) brain cells (30, 31).....even cells in the eye. (32)

Results of other scientific studies, as indicated above, confirm that increasing and maintaining a high number of circulating adult stem cells is one of the most important factors in maintaining optimum health. Research has established that the higher the number of circulating stem cells, the greater the ability of the body to heal itself. The human body depends on stem cells in the bone marrow to repair the damage caused by daily wear and tear or after an injury or illness.

As we age, our stem cell number declines. Now whether aging causes decrease in stem cells or decrease in stem cells results in aging is a question that has not yet been answered. The bottom line is we are left with fewer stem cells as we age; the decline of adult stem cells leads to slow tissue repair, lower resistance to disease, weakness of all tissues and the development of degenerative conditions. This observation is prevalent both in clinical practice as well as in daily life, and is the reason why wounds and fractures heal quickly in children as compared to older adults.

As you read in the regenerative medicine chapter, it is very exciting how we can repair a damaged organ. What would be even more exciting is the possibility that we can maintain our natural healing system strong and healthy in the first place. If we can prevent a problem from occurring, it is much better than trying to fix or treat it.

So let's do this, let's protect the healing cells that protects us. Let's keep the system, which makes us young and healthy, young and healthy. Here are some tips:

1 - Maintain optimal body weight, because as you accumulate body fat, more and more stem cells from the blood get trapped in the fat and are taken away from the pool of cells that can provide repairs.
2 - Quit smoking, as you saw above, smoking directly and indirectly hurts the replication, release and healing ability of stem cells.
3 - Eat a diet rich in anti-oxidants, Vitamin D3, E and C, to reduce oxidative stress in the body that can damage stem cells. Clinicians had known this for a long time, but lately more research studies have repeatedly shown that a majority of people have Vitamin D deficiencies. Research also showed that Vitamin D3 promotes the nerve growth factor, and other neurotropic factors that increase stem cell proliferation and activity in the brain. (34, 35) However, too much vitamin D can be toxic.

4 - Exercise regularly at moderate intensity, as it enhances healthy microenvironment of the stem cell niches, and increases release of stem cells into the blood.

5 - Sleep well in order to release a healthy dose of melatonin and growth hormone, both of which support healthy stem cell functions.

6 - Practice stress reduction activities; meditation, yoga, visualization, etc. to reduce stress, which suppresses stem cell proliferation.

7 - Maintain a healthy cholesterol level with the help of diet, exercise and statins. The last one improves stem cell activity by direct inhibition of HMG-COA reductase. Statins have been demonstrated to potently augment endothelial progenitor cell differentiation in mononuclear cells and hematopoietic stem cells. (36)

8 - Consider supplementation using fucoidan. (37,38) and AFA containing blue green algae. (39, 40) Negative effects of stress on the body can be reduced by taking supplements of N-acetyl-cysteine which is a neuro protective antioxidant. Other supplements such as a cocktail of green tea, astralagus, goji berry extracts, antioxidant ellagic acid, immune enhancer beta 1, 3 glucan and vitamin D3, in clinical studies was able to increase the number of stem cells circulating in the blood. "Hematopoietic stem cells and endothelial progenitor cells increased after taking this nutritional supplement, suggesting that the supplement may be a useful stimulator for both types of stem cells." (41)

The next time you see someone hurting their body and their health ……...........
Think.

# Conclusion

*The great enemy of the truth is very often not the lie, deliberate, contrived*
*and dishonest, but the myth, persistent, persuasive and unrealistic.*
*~John F. Kennedy*

No matter where in the world you go these days, you will find a tug of war between two unlikely opponents, two, who you would imagine and expect to be on the same side. I am talking about the clinical researchers aka, physicians and lab researchers aka, scientists. The scientists argue and insist that we do not know enough and should not yet take the stem cell treatment to patients. Many physicians and surgeons believe and support taking these treatments to clinic once we know they are safe and have enough knowledge and experience behind them to start trialing them on humans. Most of these researchers and physicians are well-meaning and highly intelligent professionals but with a very different viewpoint. (1)

So when is it too early to take a treatment to clinical trials from the lab bench? And when are we letting it wither on the vine while patients die waiting?

Let me describe it with a very relevant example from history; the discovery of Insulin. Though diabetes has been known as a disease for over 3000 years, until the discovery of insulin in 1922, there was no treatment for diabetes. Most effective management was a very strict diet, extremely restricted in sugar intake, to the point of starvation. However, this barely bought the patients a few extra months or years, and it remained a feared and lethal disease. (2)

Observation of diseased pancreas in dead, diabetic animals and humans pointed towards this organ as a likely source, but it took many more years to discover the unique part of a pancreas which secretes a substance that, if administered to animals, improves their diabetes. Experimentation on dog models of diabetes (dogs with their pancreas removed) proved that the animals get better when extracts of dry pancreata are injected in their blood.

In early1921, armed with this basic knowledge, Dr. Frederick Banting came up with the idea of isolating this pancreatic substance that can fix diabetes. In October of the same year, with his assistant, Charles Best, they managed to extract the insulin-producing islets of Langerhans from healthy dog pancreata. Working at the University of Toronto's lab in Canada, they used this extract to prove that the substance in these cells was in fact a treatment for diabetes. They named it "Insulin" after the term 'insuline', previously used to describe a hypothetical substance which controls blood sugar. With the help of a biochemist, Bertram Collip, they extracted and purified large amounts of insulin from slaughter house beef pancreata. (3)

In January 1922, Leonard Thompson, a 14-year-old Toronto boy, dying of diabetes, became the first person to receive insulin. He responded very well and from near death, rapidly regained his strength. (4) The trial was expanded to other volunteer diabetics who showed similarly positive results. The very next year's Nobel Prize for Medicine was awarded to the discovery of insulin. In the meantime pharmaceutical company Eli Lilly started mass production of porcine insulin and by mid-1923 it was widely available in North America; probably the fastest transition from concept to clinic. By the end of 1923, insulin production had crossed the Atlantic. (3)

Essentially, from the October 1921 isolation of insulin to January 1922, the first patient injection, leading to the mass production in the beginning of 1923, altogether from discovery to saving lives, insulin took less than 18 months. The questions are:

Did we know the molecular structure of insulin until 1958? No.

Did we know the mechanism of action until decades later? No.

Did we have the optimal form of the drug at the time of its first use? No.

Did we know its long term effects? Of course not.

Did it save the lives of people who definitely would have died without it? A resounding yes!

The fact is that early insulin was extracted from animals. It often caused allergic reactions. Impurities in the product caused local induration and nodules. Lack of standardization caused high and low blood sugars. Lack of long-acting form required frequent injections. The mechanism of action of insulin is very complex using a series of intracellular signals, by a variety of substances, and wasn't well understood until years later. (5) In fact even today, we don't completely understand how exactly all its functions are accomplished.

We have discovered hundreds of problems with insulin in the past 93 years and have improved insulin in hundreds of ways making it better, safer and easier to use. The first genetically engineered, synthetic "human" insulin was produced in 1978. Insulin pens became available just over a decade ago and insulin pumps only in this decade. Inhaled insulin is permeating the market now and for the first time encapsulated insulin-producing cell implants are approaching the final stages of development. I guarantee that we will continue to see improvement and new discoveries related to insulin in the coming years and decades.

Now nearly one hundred years since its discovery, do we know everything there is to know about insulin? If anyone claims we do, consider it a hyperbole, because we do not. Does that mean we should have waited until we knew the detailed mechanism of action, exact molecular structure, and complete side effect profile or until we had developed the human form of insulin, and let people die? You and I both know the answer, and insulin is not the only instance, the smallpox vaccine, penicillin, blood transfusion, heart transplant - the history of medicine is rife with similar examples.

Understanding the mechanism of action or exact molecular structure is not an absolute prerequisite. We must have respect for the value of pure empiricism in medical innovation, or we will forever be in the labs, never reaching clinics. There is only so much you can learn from animal studies, about what cells can and cannot do. The rest of the experience will have to come from their clinical application. I agree that many of the rogue clinics abroad may be selling snake oil, but there is so little being offered in the United States that people are forced to go abroad. If one is about to lose eyesight or is looking at a life in a wheelchair, who would not search for hope.

I say, shame on those who take advantage of such vulnerable people, but also shame on those who force these vulnerable people in the mouth of sharks, because the options in their own country are limited at best. (6) There should be opportunities here at home for these people, who are running out of time, or who chose to undergo experimental treatment after informed consent. Access to aggressive translational work using adult stem cells in clinical applications should be universal. There should be liberal laws for compassionate use of safe but "under study" procedures. (7) These patients should have the opportunity to get these experimental therapies in an ethical and monitored setting. (8) These programs need to be FDA-approved with rigorous research protocols so that we not only provide therapies with upward potential, but also avail occasions to learn and optimize our approaches.

Throughout this book I have made arguments against the objections to moving toward clinical use. These objections go against conventional wisdom. (9, 10) The principles of therapeutic development should form the basis of clinical trials, once adequate pre-clinical and safety information has been gathered; compassionate and experimental clinical use should proceed. For instance, hematologists have been safely using cell-based therapies for decades, so for other specialties to use the same procedure, though for alternate applications, in most cases is still safe and worthy of empirical use. This is especially true when we have hundreds of case reports, multiple studies and a growing number of professionals with first-hand experience.

There has always been a good dose of mystery in science and medicine. To wait until we understand everything about these cells, would mean we will delay for a long time the clinical use and the healing potential they carry. There is an unknown, and an unknowable, in science, and a wise scientist and clinician should be able to appreciate that difference.

It is not to say that we should ignore the risks or disregard important differences such as the ones between adult and embryonic stem cells (ESC). We may now be equipped to safely use adult stem cells but clearly not ready to clinically utilize the ESC without significant manipulation. It may be possible in the future, but not today. On the other hand, autologous adult stem cells and umbilical cord-derived stem cells are ripe for clinical practice; they have a good safety record, established application protocols and minimal risk. More clinical trials, data collection and empirical use should be encouraged to find the best mix, best source, best dose and the best method to take advantage of these amazing medics of nature that can go into a variety of disease states to wipe off inflammation, reduce immune reaction and regenerate tissues.

iPS cells also promise many benefits but just as many unknowns, they need further research and investigations as well. There are still many unanswered questions that need explanations. According to a recent report by Jeong Tae Do from Seoul University, Korea, it has come to light that initially silenced genes during the development of iPS cells can sometimes spontaneously reactivate and revert to pluripotency. This signals the risk of tumor formation, making the safety of some iPS-derived cells a concern. It also raises the question whether this effect is specific to the retroviral system, or do all iPSC-derived stem cells suffer in the same manner? (11)

Ongoing research on iPS and embryonic stem cells is imperative for learning what nature has to teach us and what may lead us to new and exciting treatment possibilities. When I contemplate the ongoing resistance to this research and the hurdles placed in the way of science, I find myself asking... should a strong viewpoint or a personal / religious belief of some people or some politicians be forced on the rest of the society?

There are millions of people, many nations, and even some major religions, who are not against the embryonic stem cell research, if the cells are derived from less than 14 day old embryos that are leftover from IVF, and destined for destruction. Under these circumstances, if we ignore the opinions of a majority of the scientists and experts in the field, then those amongst us, who have strong beliefs for or against a position, should carefully examine the dangerous precedent it sets. Let me explain...

Forget the diversity of views between major world religions; even within Christianity different sects have different views about medical care. A common example is that of Jehovah's witnesses who believe that the Bible prohibits ingesting blood, and Christians, therefore, should not donate their own blood or accept blood transfusions. Based on their religious belief, should we not have developed blood transfusion as a treatment to save lives? Or should we now stop offering it to all others even if they don't share this belief?

Similarly, there are many churches in the United States whose members firmly believe that traditional medical treatment is sinful. These groups believe that prayer not only can heal but resurrect a dead child, that there is no need for medical attention no matter how sick the child or how treatable the disease might be. They choose prayer over the services of a competent doctor so their religious beliefs take precedence over seeking medical treatment. (12, 13)

Examples include the First Century Gospel Church in Philadelphia; Church of the First Born in Albany, New York; Followers of Christ Church in Idaho, California, and Oregon, and Church of Wells in East Texas. There are hundreds more, but the reason I chose these specific ones is because all of them are associated with recent court cases where member parents let their kids die from treatable illnesses but refused to allow medical care. These kids died of conditions like diabetes, pneumonia and other treatable infections, or during attempted exorcism for autism.

In 2013, in Albany, NY, a 12-year-old girl was deprived by her parents of life-saving medical care for diabetes and died. The same year, in a Pentecostal community of the First Century Gospel Church in northeast Philadelphia, the parents of Brandon allowed him to die from pneumonia while they prayed, instead of giving him antibiotics. His brother, Kent, had died 3 years earlier under similar circumstances. In the police report the father stated, "We believe in divine healing, that Jesus shed blood for our healing and that he died on the cross to break the devil's power."

In 2012, a few days old baby Faith, of Wells, Texas, was denied medical care because the "elders" in the Church of Wells decided prayer over medicine for the new baby. As a result, Faith died of a routinely treatable condition. Followers of Christ Church in Idaho also rely on faith healing, not medicine. According to public records, 22 months old, Preston J. Bowers, died in March 2011 of pneumonia, 14-year-old Rockwell Alexander died after a two-week long respiratory illness and Pamela Jade Eells, 16, died in November 2011 of pneumonia. Arrian J.Granden, a 15-year-old, died in June 2012 suffering from food poisoning and excessive vomiting that ruptured her esophagus. I can assure you the list doesn't stop here.

Attempts to change the laws to hold these parents accountable are met with political resistance with accusations that this will trample on religious freedoms and parental rights. Followers of these churches insist that this is about the belief that God is in charge of whether the kids will live or whether they will die. Therefore, none of these children were allowed to receive medical care that would have saved their lives.

Here is my point of telling you all this. Either you believe these parents do have the right to withhold emergency medical care from their children, and let them die or you don't think that these parents should be allowed to deny sick children the right to the best medical treatment, irrespective of their own religious beliefs. If you side with the later, then who are we to deny millions of sick people the right and access to the best treatment science and medicine can offer, because of our beliefs? The view that some people hold about the status of an 8-day old embryo is not universal, just like the view of Jehovah's witnesses about transfusion is not universal or the view of the Church of the First Born about medical care is not universal. How would we feel if any one of the above views were forced upon our sick children?

These challenges are not only limited to medical care for acute illnesses. These decisions also come into play in preventive medical care. An example is the ongoing battle over Polio vaccination in Pakistan and Afghanistan or HPV (human papilloma virus) vaccination in Alberta, Canada, where, under intense pressure, Calgary's Catholic school board finally lifted a ban on administering the vaccine in its schools but a senior clergymen sent a new controversial letter to parents few months ago warning that the shots could encourage pre-marital sex. This was just as the province expanded the program to immunize both boys and girls, against the sexually transmitted virus which causes several types of cancers both in males and females. (14)

These arguments are not likely to end any time soon. It is, therefore, imperative that each one of us understands the real science and facts behind these arguments. This is the only way to reach a consensus that reflects the wishes and desires of the majority. In order to do the most good for most people, everyone needs to know what is good for them, and clearly understand the benefits, risks and ethical considerations, so that they cannot be led astray. This is the whole premise of this book. A well-informed patient is a better patient and a better consumer of healthcare.

We are already well into the exciting era of stem cells. Stem cell therapies hold great promise for the treatment of many diseases that are a major source of pain and grief. Alzheimer's disease, Parkinson's disease, Stroke, Myocardial infarction, Diabetes, Multiple sclerosis, Amyotrophic lateral-sclerosis, etc. are robbing people of a decent quality of life every day. Transplantation of specific stem cells into the injured tissue, to stimulate, replace or repair the lost or damaged cells, is a promising way to heal and cure.

The recent progress in the field of cell replacement, tissue engineering, and organ generation, is starting to give us a sneak peek into what the future of medicine may look like. Let us hope that we appreciate the significance of this revolution and realize how important it is for us and for the human race in general, and ensure that science is given an unrestricted opportunity to reach its full potential.

I hope that after reading this book you now share some of my passion and excitement about the stem cell filed in general and its promising applications in clinical practice in particular. I intend to keep writing books on topics of medical interest that are educational, informative and entertaining, so that more of us can take an active role in our health and well-being and can be an involved driver of our own healthcare.

# References

PREFACE

1 -   Gurdon, JB, Elsdale TR, Fischberg M. Sexually mature individuals of Xenopuslaevis from the transplantation of single somatic nuclei.

2 -   Till J, McCulloch E. A direct measurement of the radiation sensitivity of normal mouse bone marrow cells. Radiation Research 14 (2): 213–222, 1961.

3 -   Evans M, Kaufman M. Establishment in culture of pluripotential cells from mouse embryos. Nature 292 (5819): 154–156, 1981.

4 -   Martin G. Isolation of a pluripotent cell line from early mouse embryos cultured in medium conditioned by teratocarcinoma stem cells. ProcNatlAcadSci USA 78 (12): 7634–7638, 1981.

5 -   Campbell KHS, McWhir J, Ritchie WA, Wilmut I. Sheep cloned by nuclear transfer from a cultured cell line. Nature 380 (6569): 64–66, 1996.

6 -   Jones J, Marshall V, Swiergiel J, Waknitz M, Shapiro S, Itskovits-Eldor J, Thomson J. Embryonic stem cell lines derived from human blastocysts. Science 282 (5391): 1145–1147, 1998.

7 -   Takahashi K, Yamanaka S. Induction of pluripotent stem cells from mouse embryonic and adult fibroblast cultures by defined factors. Cell 126: 663–676, 2006.

8 -   Takahashi K, Tanabe K, Ohnuki M, Narita M, Ichisaka T, Tomoda K, Yamanaka S. Induction of pluripotent stem cells from adult human fibroblasts by defined factors. Cell 131: 861–872, 2007.

9 -   Wernig M, Zhao JP, Pruszak J, Hedlund E, Fu D, Soldner F, Broccoli V, Constantine-Paton M, Isacson O, Jaenisch R. Neurons derived from reprogrammed fibroblasts functionally integrate into the fetal brain and

improve symptoms of Parkinson's disease. Proc. Natl. Acad. Sci. USA 105(15): 5856-5861, 2008.

10 - Vierbuchen T, Ostermeier A, Pang ZP, Kokubu Y, Sudhof TC, Wernig M. Direct conversion of fibroblasts to functional neurons by defined factors. Nature 463 (7284): 1035-41. Epub 2010 Jan 27.

11 - Ieda M, Fu J, Delgado-Olguin P, Vedantham V, Hayashi Y, Bruneau B, Srivastava D. Direct reprogramming of fibroblasts into functional cardiomyocytes by defined factors. Cell 142: 375-386, 2010.

12 - Szabo E, Rampalli S, Risueno R, Schnerch A, Mitchell R, Fiebig-Comyn A, Levadoux-Martin M, Bhatia M. Direct conversion of human fibroblasts to multilineage blood progenitors. Nature 468: 521-526, 2010.

13 - Qian L, Huang Y, Spencer CI, Foley A, Vedantham V, Liu L, Conway SJ, Fu JD, Srivastava D. In vivo reprogramming of murine cardiac fibroblasts into induced cardiomyocytes. Nature 485: 593–8, 2012.

14 - Ring KL, Tong LM, Balestra ME, Javier R, Andrews-Zwilling Y, Li G, Walker D, Zhang WR, Kreitzer AC, Huang Y. Direct reprogramming of mouse and human fibroblasts into multipotent neural stem cells with a single factor. Cell Stem Cell 11: 100-9, 2012.

## CHAPTER 1 INTRODUCTION

1 - De Lacey, Lynda. Australia's Greatest Inventions (Large Print 16pt). ReadHowYouWant. com, 2010.

2 - Körbling, Martin, and ZeevEstrov. "Adult stem cells for tissue repair—a new therapeutic concept?." New England Journal of Medicine 349.6 (2003): 570-582.

3 - Lederman, Norman G., and Kenneth Tobin. "The nature of science." Dilemmas of Science Teaching: Perspectives on Problems of Practice (2002): 7.

4 - Bentley, Ronald. "The development of penicillin: genesis of a famous antibiotic." Perspectives in biology and medicine 48.3 (2005): 444-452.

5 - Rosenthal, Nadia. "Prometheus's vulture and the stem-cell promise." New England Journal of Medicine 349.3 (2003): 267-274.

6 - Mimeault, M., R. Hauke, and S. K. Batra. "Stem cells: a revolution in therapeutics—recent advances in stem cell biology and their therapeutic

applications in regenerative medicine and cancer therapies." Clinical Pharmacology & Therapeutics 82.3 (2007): 252-264.

CHAPTER 2 HISTORY OF DISEASE:

1 -   Leventi, I. Hygieia in classical Greek art. Athens, 2003

2 -   Smith, Amy C. Polis and Personification in Classical Athenian Art. Vol. 19.Brill, 2011.

3 -   Cohen, Henry."The evolution of the concept of disease." Proceedings of the Royal Society of Medicine 48.3 (1955): 155.

4 -   Davis, Audrey B. "Some implications of the circulation theory for disease theory and treatment in the seventeenth century." Journal of the history of medicine and allied sciences 26.1 (1971): 28-39.

5 -   McClusky III, David A., et al. "Tribute to a triad: history of splenic anatomy, physiology, and surgery—part 1." World journal of surgery 23.3 (1999): 311-325.

6 -   Dobrzycki, Jerzy."Nicolaus Copernicus—His Life and Work."The Scientific World of Copernicus. Springer Netherlands, 1973.13-37.

7 -   Collier, Roger. "Legumes, lemons and streptomycin: A short history of the clinical trial." Canadian Medical Association Journal 180.1 (2009): 23-24.

8 -   Bhatt, Arun. "Evolution of clinical research: a history before and beyond James Lind." Perspectives in clinical research 1.1 (2010): 6.

9 -   Riedel, Stefan."Edward Jenner and the history of smallpox and vaccination."Proceedings (Baylor University. Medical Center) 18.1 (2005): 21.

10 - Durbach N. They might as well brand us: Working class resistance to compulsory vaccination in Victorian England. The Society for the Social History of Medicine. 2000;13:45-62.)

11 - Giangrande, Paul LF."The history of blood transfusion." British Journal of Haematology 110.4 (2000): 758-767.

12 - Brown, Harcourt. "Jean Denis and Transfusion of Blood, Paris, 1667-1668." Isis (1948): 15-29.

13 - Guglielmo, Thomas A. ""Red Cross, Double Cross": Race and America's World War II-Era Blood Donor Service." The Journal of American History 97.1 (2010): 63-90.

## CHAPTER 3 THE CELL

1 - Schopf, JW (2006). Fossil evidence of Archaean life. Philos Trans R SocLond B BiolSci 29;361(1470):869-85.

2 - Ballard, J. William O., and Michael C. Whitlock. "The incomplete natural history of mitochondria." Molecular ecology 13.4 (2004): 729-744.

3 - Wilson, David S., et al. "High resolution crystal structure of a paired (Pax) class cooperative homeodomain dimer on DNA." Cell 82.5 (1995): 709-719.

4 - Wang, A. H., et al. "Molecular structure of a left-handed double helical DNA fragment at atomic resolution." Nature 282.5740 (1979): 680-686.

5 - Shay, Jerry W., and Woodring E. Wright. "Hayflick, his limit, and cellular ageing." Nature reviews Molecular cell biology 1.1 (2000): 72-76.

6 - Vaziri, Homayoun, et al. "Evidence for a mitotic clock in human hematopoietic stem cells: loss of telomeric DNA with age." Proceedings of the National Academy of Sciences 91.21 (1994): 9857-9860.

7 - Tesar, Paul J., et al. "New cell lines from mouse epiblast share defining features with human embryonic stem cells." Nature 448.7150 (2007): 196-199.

8 - Turner, D. "ES07. 02 The human leucocyte antigen (HLA) system." Voxsanguinis 87.s1 (2004): 87-90.

9 - Porcelli, Steven, et al. "Recognition of cluster of differentiation 1 antigens by human CD4– CD8>– cytolytic T lymphocyte." (1989): 447-450.

## CHAPTER 4 STEM CELL

1 - Ellison, Peter Thorpe, and Peter Thorpe Ellison. On fertile ground: A natural history of human reproduction. Harvard University Press, 2009.

2 - Hertig, A. T., et al. "Thirty four fertilized human ova, good, bad and indifferent, recovered from 210 women of un known fertility. A Study of Biologic Wastage in Early Human Pregnancy." Pediatrics 23.1 (1959): 202-211.

3 - Dunsford, I., et al. "Human blood-group chimera." British medical journal 2.4827 (1953): 81.

4 - Hipp, Jennifer, and Anthony Atala. "Sources of stem cells for regenerative medicine." Stem cell reviews 4.1 (2008): 3-11.

## CHAPTER 5 HUMAN EMBRYONIC STEM CELLS

1 - (Levenberg, S. (2002). "Endothelial cells derived from human embryonic stem cells". Proceedings of the National Academy of Sciences99 (7): 4391–4396.)

2 - Thomson, James A., et al. "Embryonic stem cell lines derived from human blastocysts." science 282.5391 (1998): 1145-1147.

3 - Dörner, Günther, et al. "Gene-and environment-dependent neuroendocrine etiogenesis of homosexuality and transsexualism." Experimental and Clinical Endocrinology & Diabetes 98.05 (1991): 141-150.

## CHAPTER 6 ADULT STEM CELL

1 - Wagers, Amy J., and Irving L. Weissman. "Plasticity of adult stem cells." Cell 116.5 (2004): 639-648.

2 - Colter, David C., Ichiro Sekiya, and Darwin J. Prockop. "Identification of a subpopulation of rapidly self-renewing and multipotential adult stem cells in colonies of human marrow stromal cells." Proceedings of the National Academy of Sciences 98.14 (2001): 7841-7845.

3 - Sakaguchi, Yusuke, et al. "Comparison of human stem cells derived from various mesenchymal tissues: superiority of synovium as a cell source." Arthritis & Rheumatism 52.8 (2005): 2521-2529.

4 - Jiang, Yuehua, et al. "Pluripotency of mesenchymal stem cells derived from adult marrow." Nature 418.6893 (2002): 41-49.

5 - Gage, Fred H. "Mammalian neural stem cells." Science 287.5457 (2000): 1433-1438.

## CHAPTER 7 UMBLICAL CORD STEM CELLS

1 - Cairo MS, Wagner JE (1997). "Placental and/or umbilical cord blood: an alternative source of hematopoietic stem cells for transplantation.".Blood90 (12): 4665–4678

2 - Hal E. Broxmeyer PhD and Franklin O. Smith MD (2009)."Cord Blood Hematopoietic Cell Transplantation.".Thomas' Hematopoietic Cell Transplantation, Fourth Edition

3 - Cord Blood for Neonatal Hypoxic-Ischemic Encephalopathy, Autologous Cord Blood Cells for Hypoxic Ischemic Encephalopathy Study 1. Phase I Study of Feasibility and Safety

4 - Haller MJ, etal.; Viener, HL; Wasserfall, C; Brusko, T; Atkinson, MA; Schatz, DA (2008). "Autologous umbilical cord blood infusion for type 1 diabetes.".Exp. Hematol.36 (6): 710–715

5 - Vendrame M, et al.; (2006). "Cord blood rescues stroke-induced changes in splenocyte phenotype and function". Exp. Neurol.199 (1): 191–200.

6 - Vendrame M, et al.; (2005). "Anti-inflammatory effects of human cord blood cells in a rat model of stroke". Stem Cells Dev.14 (5): 595–604.

7 - Duke University, Neonatal Hypoxic-Ischemic Encephalopathy; Phase I clinical trial NCT00593242,

8 - Revoltella RP, et al.; (2008). "Cochlear repair by transplantation of human cord blood CD133+ cells to nod-scid mice made deaf with kanamycin and noise". Cell Transplant.17 (6): 665–678

9 - Harris DT, et al.; (2007)."The potential of cord blood stem cells for use in regenerative medicine".ExpertOpin. Biol. Ther.7 (9): 1311–1322.

10 - Zhao Y, Wang H, Mazzone T (Aug 1, 2006). "Identification of stem cells from human umbilical cord blood with embryonic and hematopoietic characteristics".Exp Cell Res312 (13): 2454–2464

11 - Uccelli A, etal.; (2008). "Mesenchymal stem cells in health and disease.".Nature Reviews Immunology8 (9): 726–735

12 - Dominici M, etal.; (2006). "Minimal criteria for defining multipotent mesenchymal stromal cells. The International Society for Cellular Therapy position statement". Cytotherapy.8 (4): 315–317

13 - Haller, M.J.etal (2008)."Autologous umbilical cord blood infusion for type 1 diabetes".Exp. Hematol36 (6): 710–715.

14 - De Coppi P, et al "Isolation of amniotic stem cell lines with potential for therapy". (2007). Nature Biotechnology25 (5): 100–106.

## CHAPTER 8 INDUCED PLURIPOTENT STEM CELLS (iPSc)

1 - Okita, Keisuke, Tomoko Ichisaka, and Shinya Yamanaka. "Generation of germline-competent induced pluripotent stem cells." Nature 448.7151 (2007): 313-317.

2 -   Yu, Junying, et al. "Induced pluripotent stem cell lines derived from human somatic cells." Science 318.5858 (2007): 1917-1920.

3 -   Tapscott, Stephen J., et al. "MyoD1: a nuclear phosphoprotein requiring a Myc homology region to convert fibroblasts to myoblasts." Science 242.4877 (1988): 405-411.

4 -   Yamanaka, Shinya. "A fresh look at iPS cells." Cell 137.1 (2009): 13-17.

5 -   Kathrin Meyer et al Direct conversion of patient fibroblasts demonstrates non-cell autonomous toxicity of astrocytes to motor neurons in familial and sporadic ALS PNASJanuary 14, 2014vol. 111 no. 2 829-832

6 -   Szabo E, Rampalli S, Risueno R, Schnerch A, Mitchell R, Fiebig-Comyn A, Levadoux-Martin M, Bhatia M. Direct conversion of human fibroblasts to multilineage blood progenitors. Nature 2010. 468:521–526.

7 -   Jin Z, Okamoto S, Osakada F, Homma K, Assawachananont J, Hirami Y, Iwata T, Takahashi M. Modeling retinal degeneration using patient-specific induced pluripotent stem cells. PLoS On. 2011 Feb 10;6(2):e17084.

8 -   Tsuji O, et al Therapeutic potential of appropriately evaluated safe-induced pluripotent stem cells for spinal cord injury. ProcNatlAcad Sci. USA, 2010, 107:12704–12709, Epub 6 Jul 2010

9 -   Efe JA, Hilcove S, Kim J, Zhou H, Ouyang K, Wang G, Chen J, Ding S. Conversion of mouse fibroblasts into cardiomyocytes using a direct reprogramming strategy. Nature 2012, 485, 593–598

10 -  Qian L, Huang Y, Spencer CI, Foley A, Vedantham V, Liu L, Conway SJ, Fu JD, Srivastava D. In vivo reprogramming of murine cardiac fibroblasts into induced cardiomyocytes. Nature. 2012, 485:593–598.

11 -  Song B, Smink A, Jones C, Callaghan J, Firth S, Bernard C, Laslett A, Kerr P, Ricardo S. The directed differentiation of human iPS cells into kidney podocytes. PLoS ONE 7(9): e46453.

12 -  Rashid ST, et al Modeling inherited metabolic disorders of the liver using human induced pluripotent stem cells. J Clin Invest. 2010, 120: 3127–3136

13 -  Jeon K, et al. Differentiation and transplantation of functional pancreatic beta cells generated from induced pluripotent stem cells derived from a type 1 diabetes mouse model. Stem Cells and Development. 2012, 21:2642–2655

14 - Hiramatsu K, et al Generation of hyaline cartilaginous tissue from mouse adult dermal fibroblast culture by defined factors. J Clin Invest. 2011 121: 640–657, Epub: 10 Jan 2011.

15 - Medvedev SP, et al. Human induced pluripotent stem cells derived from fetal neural stem cells successfully undergo directed differentiation into cartilage. Stem Cells Devel. 2011, 20: 1099–1112, Epub 17 Oct 2010.

## CHAPTER 9 ETHICS AND STEM CELLS

1 - Kennedy, Randall. "How Are We Doing with Loving: Race, Law, and Intermarriage." BUL Rev. 77 (1997): 815.

2 - Thomas, Kendall. "The Eclipse of Reason: A Rhetorical Reading of Bowers v. Hardwick." Virginia Law Review (1993): 1805-1832.

3 - Trosino, James. "American Wedding: Same-Sex Marriage and the Miscegenation Analogy." BUL Rev. 73 (1993): 93.

4 - James Hastings (ed), Encyclopaedia of Religion and Ethics (1971) vol viii at 445 ('Marriage (Greek').

5 - Dembitz, Nanette. "Racial Discrimination and the Military Judgment: The Supreme Court's Korematsu and Endo Decisions." Columbia Law Review (1945): 175-239.

6 - Richey, Warren (December 5, 2007). "Key Guantánamo cases hit Supreme Court". The Christian Science Monitor.

7 - Bruinius, Harry (2007). Better for All the World: The Secret History of Forced Sterilization and America's Quest for Racial Purity. New York: Vintage Books.

8 - Kühl, Stefan (2002-02-14). The Nazi Connection: Eugenics, American Racism, and German National Socialism. p. 86

9 - Ziegler, Mary (2008). "Eugenic Feminism: Mental Hygiene, The Women's Movement, And The Campaign For Eugenic Legal Reform, 1900-1935". Harvard Journal of Law & Gender 31 (1): 211–236

10 - Final Report of the Tuskegee Syphilis Study Legacy Committee". Tuskegee Syphilis Study Legacy Committee. 1996-05-20

11 - Katz RV, Kegeles SS, Kressin NR, et al. (November 2006). "The Tuskegee Legacy Project: willingness of minorities to participate in biomedical research". J Health Care Poor Underserved 17 (4): 698–715

12 - Levran, David, et al. "Prospective evaluation of blastocyst stage transfer vs. zygote intrafallopian tube transfer in patients with repeated implantation failure." Fertility and sterility 77.5 (2002): 971-977.

13 - Truog, Robert D., and Walter M. Robinson. "Role of brain death and the dead-donor rule in the ethics of organ transplantation." Critical care medicine 31.9 (2003): 2391-2396.

14 - Jacobs, P.A. (1990) The role of chromosome abnormalities in reproductive failure. Reprod. Nutr. Dev., (Suppl. 1), 63s-74s)

15 - Spahn, Elizabeth, and Barbara Andrade. "Mis-Conceptions: The Moment of Conception in Religion, Science, and Law." USFL Rev. 32 (1997): 261.

16 - Robertson, John A. "Human embryonic stem cell research: ethical and legal issues." Nature Reviews Genetics 2.1 (2001): 74-78.

17 - Robertson, John A. "Extending preimplantation genetic diagnosis: the ethical debate Ethical issues in new uses of preimplantation genetic diagnosis." Human Reproduction 18.3 (2003): 465-471.

18 - Olanow, C. Warren, et al. "A double-blind controlled trial of bilateral fetal nigral transplantation in Parkinson's disease." Annals of neurology 54.3 (2003): 403-414.

19 - Steinbock, Bonnie. Life before birth: the moral and legal status of embryos and fetuses. Oxford University Press, 2011.

## CHAPTER 10 VIRGIN BIRTH to HUMAN CLONING

1 - Steinbock, Bonnie. "Reproductive Cloning: Another Look." U. Chi. Legal F. (2006): 87.

2 - French, Andrew J., Samuel H. Wood, and Alan O. Trounson. "Human therapeutic cloning (NTSC)." Stem cell reviews 2.4 (2006): 265-276.

3 - Tomlinson, J. "The advantages of hermaphroditism and parthenogenesis." Journal of Theoretical Biology 11.1 (1966): 54-58.

4 - De Lafayette, Maximillien. Ba'ab: The Anunnaki Stargate. Lulu. com, 2010.

5 - Sitchin, Zecharia. The Lost Book of Enki: Memoirs and Prophecies of an Extraterrestrial God. Inner Traditions/Bear & Co, 2004.

6 - Sitchin, Zecharia. The King who Refused to Die: The Anunnaki and the Search for Immortality. Inner Traditions/Bear & Co, 2013.

7 -   Illmensee, Karl, Peter C. Hoppe, and Carlo M. Croce. "Chimeric mice derived from human—mouse hybrid cells." Proceedings of the National Academy of Sciences 75.4 (1978): 1914-1918.

8 -   Wilmut, Ian, Keith Campbell, and Colin Tudge. The second creation: Dolly and the age of biological control. Harvard University Press, 2001.

9 -   Alcíbar, Miguel. "Human Cloning and the Raelians Media Coverage and the Rhetoric of Science." Science Communication 30.2 (2008): 236-265.

10 -  Wurm, Florian M. "Production of recombinant protein therapeutics in cultivated mammalian cells." Nature biotechnology 22.11 (2004): 1393-1398.

11 -  Colman, Alan, and Alexander Kind. "Therapeutic cloning: concepts and practicalities." Trends in biotechnology 18.5 (2000): 192-196.

## CHAPTER 11 HYBRID, CYBRID and CHIMERAS

1 -   Schmitt, Marilyn Low. "Bellerophon and the Chimaera in Archaic Greek Art." American Journal of Archaeology (1966): 341-347.

2 -   Mayo, Margaret. Mythical Birds and Beasts from Many Lands. Dutton Books, 1997.

3 -   Hogan, Brigid, Frank Costantini, and Elizabeth Lacy. Manipulating the mouse embryo: a laboratory manual. Vol. 34. Cold Spring Harbor, NY: Cold spring harbor laboratory, 1986.

4 -   Szymkowiak, Eugene J., and Ian M. Sussex. "What chimeras can tell us about plant development." Annual review of plant biology 47.1 (1996): 351-376.

5 -   Landy, H. J., and L. G. Keith. "The vanishing twin: a review." Human reproduction update 4.2 (1998): 177-183.

6 -   Rinkevich, B. "Human natural chimerism: an acquired character or a vestige of evolution?." Human immunology 62.6 (2001): 651-657.

7 -   Ellstrand, Norman C., Richard Whitkus, and Loren H. Rieseberg. "Distribution of spontaneous plant hybrids." Proceedings of the National Academy of Sciences 93.10 (1996): 5090-5093.

8 -   Strelchenko, Nick, et al. "Reprogramming of human somatic cells by embryonic stem cell cytoplast." Reproductive biomedicine online 12.1 (2006): 107-111.

9 -    Byrne, J., et al. "Producing primate embryonic stem cells by somatic cell nuclear transfer." Nature 450.7168 (2007).

10 -   Homer, Hayden, and Melanie Davies. "The science and ethics of human admixed embryos." Obstetrics, Gynaecology& Reproductive Medicine 19.9 (2009): 235-239.

## CHAPTER 12 HEALING IS AN INSIDE JOB

1 -    Chalfie, Martin, and Douglas Prasher. "Green fluorescent protein." U.S. Patent No. 6,146,826. 14 Nov. 2000.

2 -    Persons, Derek A., et al. "Use of the green fluorescent protein as a marker to identify and track genetically modified hematopoietic cells." Nature medicine 4.10 (1998): 1201-1205.

3 -    Terada, Naohiro, et al. "Bone marrow cells adopt the phenotype of other cells by spontaneous cell fusion." Nature 416.6880 (2002): 542-545.

4 -    Jung, Steffen, et al. "Analysis of fractalkine receptor CX3CR1 function by targeted deletion and green fluorescent protein reporter gene insertion." Molecular and cellular biology 20.11 (2000): 4106-4114.

5 -    Addington CP, et al. The role of SDF-1α-ECM crosstalk in determining neural stem cell fate. Biomaterials, 2014 Mar

6 -    Lim TC, Rokkappanavar et al Chemotactic recruitment of adult neural progenitor cells into multifunctional hydrogels providing sustained SDF-1α release and compatible structural support. FASEB J. 2013 Mar; 27(3): 1023-33

7 -    Niswander LM, et al. SDF-1 dynamically mediates megakaryocyte niche occupancy and thrombopoiesis at steady state and following radiation injury. Blood, 2014 Jul 10.

8 -    Hsieh, Patrick CH, et al. "Evidence from a genetic fate-mapping study that stem cells refresh adult mammalian cardiomyocytes after injury." Nature medicine 13.8 (2007): 970-974.

9 -    Herzog, Erica L., Li Chai, and Diane S. Krause. "Plasticity of marrow-derived stem cells." Blood 102.10 (2003): 3483-3493.

10 -   (Krause, D.S., Theise, N.D., Collector, M.I., Henegariu, O., Hwang, S., Gardner, R., Neutzel, S., and Sharkis, S.J. (2001). Multi-organ, multi-lineage engraftment by a single bone marrow-derived stem cell. Cell. 105, 369–377.)

11 - Deb, Arjun, et al. "Bone Marrow–Derived Cardiomyocytes Are Present in Adult Human Heart A Study of Gender-Mismatched Bone Marrow Transplantation Patients." Circulation 107.9 (2003): 1247-1249.

12 - Bensinger, W. I., et al. "Transplantation of allogeneic peripheral blood stem cells mobilized by recombinant human granulocyte colony-stimulating factor [see comments]." Blood 85.6 (1995): 1655-1658.

13 - Thiele J, Varus E, Wickenhauser C, et al. (2004) Mixed chimerism of cardiomyocytes and vessels after allogeneic bone marrow and stem-cell transplantation in comparison with cardiac allografts. Transplantation 77(12):1902-5.

14 - Quaini F, Urbanek K, Beltrami AP, et al. (2002) Chimerism of of the transplanted heart N Engl J Med. 346(1):5-15.

15 - Theise ND, Nimmakayalu M, Gardner R, et al. (2000) Liver from bone marrow in humans. Hepatology. 32(l):ll-6.

16 - Poulsom R, Forbes SJ, Hodivala-Dilke K, et al. (2001) Bone marrow contributes to renal parenchymal turnover and regeneration. J Pathol. 195(2):229-35.

17 - Suratt BT, Cool CD, Serls AE, et al. (2003) Human pulmonary chimerism after hematopoietic stem cell transplantation. Am.JRespir. Crit. Care Med. 168(3):318-22.

18 - Deb A, Wang S, Skelding KA, et al. (2003) Bone marrow-derived cardiomyocytes are present in adult human heart: A study of gender-mismatched bone marrow transplantation patients. Circulation 107(9):1247-9.

19 - Mezey E, Key S, Vogelsang G, et al. (2003) Transplanted bone marrow generates new neurons in human brains. Proc. Natl. Acad. Sci. USA 100, 1364-1369.

20 - Jang YY, Collector MI, Baylin SB, et al. (2004) Hematopoietic stem cells convert into liver cells within days without fusion. Nature Cell. Biol. 6(6):532-529.

21 - Pittenger, Mark F., et al. "Multilineage potential of adult human mesenchymal stem cells." science 284.5411 (1999): 143-147.

22 - Engelmann, Markus G., et al. "Autologous Bone Marrow Stem Cell Mobilization Induced by Granulocyte Colony-Stimulating Factor After Subacute ST-Segment Elevation Myocardial Infarction Undergoing Late

Revascularization Final Results From the G-CSF-STEMI Trial." Journal of the American College of Cardiology 48.8 (2006): 1712-1721.

23 - Petit, Isabelle, et al. "G-CSF induces stem cell mobilization by decreasing bone marrow SDF-1 and up-regulating CXCR4." Nature immunology 3.7 (2002): 687-694.

24 - Orlic, Donald, et al. "Mobilized bone marrow cells repair the infarcted heart, improving function and survival." Proceedings of the National Academy of Sciences 98.18 (2001): 10344-10349.

25 - Sprigg, Nikola, et al. "Granulocyte-Colony–Stimulating Factor Mobilizes Bone Marrow Stem Cells in Patients With Subacute Ischemic Stroke The Stem Cell Trial of Recovery EnhanceMent After Stroke (STEMS) Pilot Randomized, Controlled Trial (ISRCTN 16784092)." Stroke 37.12 (2006): 2979-2983.

26 - Kucia, Magda, et al. "Tissue-specific muscle, neural and liver stem/progenitor cells reside in the bone marrow, respond to an SDF-1 gradient and are mobilized into peripheral blood during stress and tissue injury." Blood Cells, Molecules, and Diseases 32.1 (2004): 52-57.

27 - Forrester, James S., Matthew J. Price, and Raj R. Makkar. "Stem cell repair of infarcted myocardium an overview for clinicians." Circulation 108.9 (2003): 1139-1145.

28 - Wang, Yongzhong, et al. "Changes in circulating mesenchymal stem cells, stem cell homing factor, and vascular growth factors in patients with acute ST elevation myocardial infarction treated with primary percutaneous coronary intervention." Heart 92.6 (2006): 768-774.

29 - Tomoda, Haruo, and Naoto Aoki. "Bone marrow stimulation and left ventricular function in acute myocardial infarction." Clinical cardiology 26.10 (2003): 455-457.

30 - Wollert, Kai C., and Helmut Drexler. "Clinical applications of stem cells for the heart." Circulation research 96.2 (2005): 151-163.

31 - Yip, Hon-Kan, et al. "Level and value of circulating endothelial progenitor cells in patients after acute ischemic stroke." Stroke 39.1 (2008): 69-74.

## CHAPTER 13 BONE MARROW TRANSPLANTS

1 - Santos, G. W. "History of bone marrow transplantation." Clinics in haematology 12.3 (1983): 611-639.

2 - Dausset, Jean, and Felix T. Rapaport. "THE ROLE OF BLOOD GROUP ANTIGENS IN HUMAN HISTOCOMPATIBILITY*." Annals of the New York Academy of Sciences 129.1 (1966): 408-420.

3 - Siminoff, Laura A., et al. "Public policy governing organ and tissue procurement in the United StatesResults from the National Organ and Tissue Procurement Study." Annals of Internal Medicine 123.1 (1995): 10-17.

4 - Korngold, Robert. "Biology of graft-vs.-host disease." Journal of Pediatric Hematology/Oncology 15.1 (1993): 18-27.

5 - Martin, P. J., et al. "Prochymal improves response rates in patients with steroid-refractory acute graft versus host disease (SR-GVHD) involving the liver and gut: results of a randomized, placebo-controlled, multicenter phase III trial in GVHD." Biology of Blood and Marrow Transplantation 16.2 (2010): S169-S170.

6 - Ringdén, Olle, et al. "Mesenchymal stem cells for treatment of therapy-resistant graft-versus-host disease." Transplantation 81.10 (2006): 1390-1397.

7 - Coleman, Sydney R. "Facial recontouring with lipostructure." Clinics in plastic surgery 24.2 (1997): 347-367.

8 - Sittinger, M., et al. "Tissue engineering and autologous transplant formation: practical approaches with resorbable biomaterials and new cell culture techniques." Biomaterials 17.3 (1996): 237-242.

9 - Weiss, Mark L., et al. "Immune Properties of Human Umbilical Cord Wharton's Jelly-Derived Cells." Stem cells 26.11 (2008): 2865-2874.

10 - Aggarwal, Sudeepta, and Mark F. Pittenger. "Human mesenchymal stem cells modulate allogeneic immune cell responses." Blood 105.4 (2005): 1815-1822.

11 - Heylighen, Francis. "Occam's razor." Principia cybernetica web (1997).

12 - Eisenhower, Dwight D. "Farewell Address, January 17, 1961." Public Papers of the Presidents: Dwight D. Eisenhower 61 (1960).

## CHAPTER 14 REGENERATIVE MEDICINES

1 - Fujisawa, Toshitaka. "Hydra regeneration and epitheliopeptides." Developmental dynamics 226.2 (2003): 182-189.

2 - Lewmark, P. A., and Alvarado, A. S. Bromodeoxyuridine specifically labels the regenerative stem cells of planarians. 2000). Dev Biol 220, 142-153.

3 - Saló, Emili. "The power of regeneration and the stem-cell kingdom: freshwater planarians (Platyhelminthes)." Bioessays 28.5 (2006): 546-559.

4 - Harris DT, et al.; Badowski, Michael; Ahmad, Nafees; Gaballa, Mohamed A (2007). "The potential of cord blood stem cells for use in regenerative medicine". Expert Opin. Biol. Ther.7 (9): 1311–1322

## CHAPTER 15 TISSUE ENGINEERING

1 - Mayr, Ernst. The Growth of Biological Thought. Cambridge, Massachusetts and London, England: Belknap Press, 1982.

2 - Virchow R. Die Cellular-Pathologie in ihrerBegründung auf physiologische und pathologischeGewebelehre. Berlin, Germany:A. Hirschwald; 1858.

3 - Amit M, Carpenter MK, Inokuma MS, et al. Clonally derived human embryonic stem cell lines maintain pluripotency and proliferative potential for prolonged periods of culture. Dev Biol. 2000;227(2):271-278.

4 - Park SN, Lee HJ, Lee KH, Suh H. Biological characterization of EDC-crosslinked collagen-hyaluronic acid matrix in dermal tissue restoration. Biomaterials. 2003;24(9):1631-1641.

5 - LodishH,BaltimoreD,Darnell JE. Multicellularity: cell-cell and cell-matrix interactions. In:Tenney S, ed. Molecular Cell Biology. 3rd ed. New York,NY:WH Freeman; 1995

6 - Bilodeau K, Mantovani D. Bioreactors for tissue engineering: focus on mechanical constraints. A comparative review. Tissue Eng. 2006;12(8):2367-2383.

7 - Badylak SF, Taylor D, Uygun K: Whole-organ tissue engineering: decellularization and recellularization of three-dimensional matrix scaffolds. Annu Rev Biomed Eng 2011, 13:27-53.

8 - David Y. Fozdar, Shaochen Chen et al Three-Dimensional Polymer Constructs Exhibiting a Tunable Negative Poisson's Ratio. Advanced Functional Materials, 2011.

9 - University of Arkansas, Fayetteville. "Engineered muscle-mimic research: Technique uses living cells to build engineered muscle tissue."

10 - ScienceDaily, 24 June 2014.Stem cells and pluripotent cells have been successfully used to make bone in the lab, which is compatible with surgical use in patients.

CHAPTER 16 CONCEPTS TO CLINIC: Part I

1 - Centers for Disease Control and Prevention. The State of Aging and Health in America 2013. Atlanta, GA: Centers for Disease Control and Prevention, US Dept of Health and Human Services; 2013.

2 - Satariano WA, Guralnik JM, Jackson RJ, Marottoli RA, Phelan EA, Prohaska TR. Mobioity and aging: new directions for public health action. Am J Public Health. 2012;102(8):1508-1515.

3 - Glass TA, Balfour JL. Neighborhoods, aging, and functional limitations. In: Kawachi I, Berkman LF, eds. Neighborhoods and Health. New York, NY: Oxford University Press; 2003:303-334.

4 - Atlanta Regional Commissions, Older Adults in the Atlanta Region: Preference, Practices and Potential of the 55+ Population. Atlanta, GA: Atlanta Regional Commission; 2007.

5 - Centers for Disease Control and Prevention. National Diabetes Statistics Report: Estimates of Diabetes and Its Burden in the United States, 2014. Atlanta, GA: US Department of Health and Human Services; 2014.

6 - Alzheimer's & Dementia: The Journal of the Alzheimer's AssociationVolume 10, Issue 2, Pages e47–e92, March 2014

7 - Parkinson's Disease Foundation. General information

8 - Zhang X, et al. Multilevel regression and post-stratification for small area estimation of population health outcomes: a case study of chronic obstructive pulmonary disease prevalence using BRFSS. Am J Epidemiol. 2014;179(8):1025-1033.

9 - Asthma Facts—CDC's National Asthma Control Program Grantees. Atlanta, GA: U.S. Department of Health and Human Services, Centers for Disease Control and Prevention, 2013.

10 - U.S. Cancer Statistics Working Group. United States Cancer Statistics: 1999–2011 Incidence and Mortality Web-based Report. Atlanta: U.S. DHHS, CDC and National Cancer Institute; 2014.

11 - Faul M, Xu L, Wald MM, Coronado VG. Traumatic Brain Injury in the United States: Emergency Department Visits, Hospitalizations and Deaths 2002–2006. Centers for Disease Control and Prevention, 2010

12 - Chronic Kidney Disease Surveillance System. Atlanta, GA: Centers for Disease Control and Prevention, US Dept of Health and Human Services; 2011.

13 - Lakatos PL. Recent trends in the epidemiology of inflammatory bowel diseases: up or down? World J Gastroenterol2006;12(38):6102–08.

14 - www.cdc.gov/hiv/library/reports/surveillance/2011/surveillance_ Report_ vol_23.

15 - Helmick CG, et al. Estimates of the prevalence of arthritis and other rheumatic conditions in the United States- Part I. Arthritis & Rheum. 2008: 58(1):15-25

16 - Lawrence RC, et al. Estimates of the prevalence of arthritis and other rheumatic conditions in the United States- Part II. Arthritis & Rheum. 2008: 58(1):26-35.

17 - One Degree of Separation: Paralysis and Spinal Cord Injury in the United States

18 - Olaf Bergmann and Jonas Frisén et al Evidence for Cardiomyocyte Renewal in Humans 2009, Science 324, 98 (2009)

19 - Elisa Messina, et al Isolation and Expansion of Adult Cardiac Stem Cells From Human and Murine Heart Circ. Res. 2004;95;911-921

20 - Bolli, R.et al. Cardiac stem cells in patients with ischemic cardiomyopathy (SCIPIO): initial results of a randomized phase 1 trial (2011).Lancet378, 1847–1857

21 - JozefBartunek, Cardiopoietic Stem Cell Therapy in Heart Failure: The C-CURE (Cardiopoietic stem Cell therapy in heart failure) Multicenter Randomized Trial With Lineage-Specified Biologics; 2013, Journal of the American College of Cardiology Pages 2329–2338

23 - R. Bolli, at al Cardiac stem cells in patients with ischemic cardiomyopathy (SCIPIO): initial results of a randomized phase 1 trial 2011 Lancet pp. 1847–1857

24 - R.R. Makkar at al Intracoronarycardiosphere-derived cells for heart regeneration after myocardial infarction (CADUCEUS): a prospective, randomized phase 1 trial Lancet, (2012), pp. 895–904

25 - V. Schächinger et al Improved clinical outcome after intracoronary administration of bone-marrow-derived progenitor cells in acute myocardial infarction: final 1-year results of the REPAIR-AMI trial (2006), Eur Heart J, pp. 2775–2783

26 - Deng ZR, Yang C, Ma AQ et al. 2006, Dynamic changes of plasma VEGF, SDF-1 and peripheral CD34+ cells in patients with acute myocardial infarction. Nan Fang Yi Ke Da XueXueBao26, 1637–1640.

27 - Nikos Werner, M.D et al; Circulating Endothelial Progenitor Cells and Cardiovascular Outcomes; N Engl J Med 2005; 353:999-1007

28 - Vasa M, Fichtlscherer S, Aicher A, et al. (2001) Number and migratory activity of circulating endothelial progenitor cells inversely correlate with risk factors for coronary artery disease. Circ. Res. 89:e1-e7

29 - Boomsma RA, Swaminathan PD, Geenen DL et al. 2006 Intravenously injected mesenchymal stem cells home to viablemyocardium after coronary occlusion and preserve systolic function without altering infarct size. International Journal ofCardiology122, 17–28.

30 - Li ZQ, et al. 2007 The clinical study of autologous peripheral blood stem cell transplantation by intracoronary infusion in patients with acute myocardial infarction (AMI). International Journal of Cardiology 115, 52–56.

31 - Briguori C, Reimers B, Sarais C et al. 2006 Direct intra-myocardial percutaneous delivery of autologous bone marrow in patients with refractory myocardial angina. American Heart Journal 151, 674–680.

32 - Obradovic S, Rusovic S, Balint B et al. 2004 Autologous bone marrow-derived progenitor cell transplantation for myocardialregeneration after acute infarction. Vojnosanit Pregl 61, 519–529.

33 - Ghen MJ, Roshan R, Roshan RO et al. 2006 Potential clinical applications using stem cells derived from human umbilical cord blood. Reproductive BioMedicine Online 13, 562–572.

34 - Georgina M. Ellison, et al. Adult c-kitpos Cardiac Stem Cells Are Necessary and Sufficient for Functional Cardiac Regeneration and Repair. Cell, 2013; 154 (4): 827

35 - D.M. Clifford, S.A. Fisher, S.A. Brunskill, et al. Stem cell treatment for acute myocardial infarction (2012 Feb 15), Cochrane Database Syst Rev, 2

36 - Chen SL, Fang WW, Qian J et al. 2004 Improvement of cardiac function after transplantation of autologous bone marrowmesenchymal stem cells

in patients with acute myocardial infarction. Chinese Medical Journal 117, 1443–1448.

37 - Berry MF, Engler AJ, Woo WJ et al. 2006 Mesenchymal stem cell injection after myocardial infarction improves myocardial compliance. American Journal of Physiology Heart and Circulatory Physiology.290, H2196–H2203.

38 - Fernandez-Aviles F, San Roman JA, García-Frade J et al. 2004 Experimental and clinical regenerative capability of human bonemarrow cells after myocardial infarction. Circulation Research 9, 742–748.

39 - Guo J, Lin GS, Bao CY et al. 2007 Anti-inflammation role for mesenchymal stem cells transplantation in myocardial infarction. Inflammation30, 97–104

40 - Kinkaid HY, Huang XP, Li RK, Weisel RD. What's new in cardiac cell therapy? Allogeneic bone marrow stromal cells as 'universal donor cells'.J. Card. Surg.25(3),359–366 (2010)

41 - Ptaszek LM, Mansour M, Ruskin JN, Chien KR. Towards regenerative therapy for cardiac disease. Lancet379,933–942 (2012)

42 - Caspi, O.et al.Transplantation of human embryonic stem cell-derived cardiomyocytes improves myocardial performance in infarcted rat hearts. J. Am. Coll. Cardiol.50,1884–1893 (2007)

43 - James J. H. et al; Human embryonic-stem-cell-derived cardiomyocytes regenerate non-human primate hearts. 2014;Nature510,273–277

44 - Nagaya N, Kangawa K, Itoh T et al. 2005 Transplantation of mesenchymal stem cells improves cardiac function in a rat model of dilated cardiomyopathy. Circulation 112, 1128–1135.

45 - Georgina M. Ellison, et al. Adult c-kitpos Cardiac Stem CellsAre Necessary and Sufficient for Functional Cardiac Regeneration and Repair. Cell, 2013; 154 (4): 827

46 - Briguori C, Reimers B, Sarais C et al. 2006 Direct intramyocardial percutaneous delivery of autologous bone marrow in patients with refractory myocardial angina. American Heart Journal 151, 674–680.

47 - Chen SL, Fang WW, Qian J et al. 2004 Improvement of cardiac function after transplantation of autologous bone marrow mesenchymal stem cells in patients with acute myocardial infarction. Chinese Medical Journal 117, 1443–1448.

CHAPTER 17 CONCEPTS TO CLINIC: Part II

1 - Lage, José Manuel Martínez. "100 Years of Alzheimer's disease (1906-2006)." Journal of Alzheimer's Disease 9 (2006): 15-26.

2 - Hebert LE, Weuve J, Scherr PA, Evans DA. Alzheimer disease in the United States (2010-2050) estimated using the 2010 Census. Neurology 2013;80(19):1778–83.

3 - Simard, A. R., and S. Rivest. "Neuroprotective properties of the innate immune system and bone marrow stem cells in Alzheimer's disease." Molecular psychiatry 11.4 (2006): 327-335.

4 - Blurton-Jones, Mathew, et al. "Neural stem cells improve cognition via BDNF in a transgenic model of Alzheimer disease." Proceedings of the National Academy of Sciences 106.32 (2009): 13594-13599.

5 - Lee, Hyun Ju, et al. "The therapeutic potential of human umbilical cord blood-derived mesenchymal stem cells in Alzheimer's disease." Neuroscience letters 481.1 (2010): 30-35.

6 - Lindvall, Olle, and ZaalKokaia. "Stem cells in human neurodegenerative disorders—time for clinical translation?." The Journal of clinical investigation 120.1 (2010): 29-40.

7 - De Lau, L. M. L., et al. "Incidence of parkinsonism and Parkinson disease in a general population The Rotterdam Study." Neurology 63.7 (2004): 1240-1244.

8 - Marsden, C. David, and C. Warren Olanow. "The causes of Parkinson's disease are being unraveled and rational neuroprotective therapy is close to reality." Annals of neurology 44.S1 (1998): S189-S196.

9 - Olanow, C. Warren, Jose A. Obeso, and FabrizioStocchi. "Continuous dopamine-receptor treatment of Parkinson's disease: scientific rationale and clinical implications." The Lancet Neurology 5.8 (2006): 677-687.

10 - Kim, Jong-Hoon, et al. "Dopamine neurons derived from embryonic stem cells function in an animal model of Parkinson's disease." Nature 418.6893 (2002): 50-56.

11 - Freed CR, Greene PE, Breeze RE, et al. Transplantation of embryonic dopamine neurons for severe Parkinson's disease. N Engl J Med. 2001;344(10):710-719.

12 - Hallett et al., Long-Term Health of Dopaminergic Neuron Transplants in Parkinson's Disease Patients, Cell Reports (June 5, 2014),

13 - Mendez I, Viñuela A, Astradsson A, et al. Dopamine neurons implanted into people with Parkinson's disease survive without pathology for 14 years. Nat Med. 2008;14(5):507-509.

14 - Dyment DA, Ebers GC, Sadovnick AD (February 2004). "Genetics of multiple sclerosis". Lancet Neurol 3 (92): 104–10

15 - Marrie RA (December 2004). "Environmental risk factors in multiple sclerosis aetiology". Lancet Neurol 3 (12): 709–18.

16 - McDonald, W. Ian, et al. "Recommended diagnostic criteria for multiple sclerosis: guidelines from the International Panel on the diagnosis of multiple sclerosis." Annals of neurology 50.1 (2001): 121-127.

17 - Sharma, Ratti Ram, et al. "Mesenchymal stem or stromal cells: a review of clinical applications and manufacturing practices." Transfusion 54.5 (2014): 1418-1437.

18 - GL Mancardi et al. Autologous haematopoietic stem cell transplantation with an intermediate intensity conditioning regimen in multiple sclerosis: the Italian multi-center experience, Clinical Neurology June 2012 vol. 18835-842

19 - Bing Chen et al Long-term efficacy of autologous hematopoietic stem cell transplantation in multiple sclerosis at a single institution in China; Neurological Sciences; August 2012, Volume 33, Issue 4, pp 881-886

20 - Jury L. Shevchenko et al Autologous hematopoietic stem cell transplantation with reduced-intensity conditioning in multiple sclerosis; Experimental HematologyVolume 40, Issue 11, Pages 892–898, November 2012

21 - Borchelt, David R., et al. "Superoxide dismutase 1 with mutations linked to familial amyotrophic lateral sclerosis possesses significant activity." Proceedings of the National Academy of Sciences 91.17 (1994): 8292-8296.

22 - Traynor, Bryan J., et al. "Clinical features of amyotrophic lateral sclerosis according to the El Escorial and Airlie House diagnostic criteria: a population-based study." Archives of neurology 57.8 (2000): 1171-1176.

23 - Miller, Robert G., et al. "Riluzole for amyotrophic lateral sclerosis (ALS)/ motor neuron disease (MND)." Cochrane Database Syst Rev 1.1 (2007).

24 - Eva L. Feldman MD, PhD et al; Intraspinal neural stem cell transplantation in amyotrophic lateral sclerosis: Phase 1 trial outcomes; Annals of Neurology Volume 75, Issue 3, pages 363–373, March 2014

25 - Xu Let al Human neural stem cell grafts in the spinal cord of SOD1 transgenic rats: differentiation and structural integration into the segmental motor circuitry. J Comp Neurol. 2009 Jun 1;514(4):297-309.

26 - Joyce, Nanette, et al. "Mesenchymal stem cells for the treatment of neurodegenerative disease." Regenerative medicine 5.6 (2010): 933-946.

27 - Aboody, Karen, et al. "Translating stem cell studies to the clinic for CNS repair: current state of the art and the need for a Rosetta Stone." Neuron 70.4 (2011): 597-613.

28 - Garrison FH. History of Neurology. Revised and enlarged by McHenry LC Jr. Springfield, Ill: Charles C Thomas Publishing; 1969.

29 - Roger, V.; Go, A.; Lloyd-Jones, S.; Benjamin, E.; Berry, J.; Borden, W.; Bravata, D.; Dai, S.; Ford, E.; Fox, C.; et al. Heart disease and stroke statistics—2012 update: A report from the american heart association. Circulation 2012, 125, e2–e220.

30 - Hermann DM et al; Promoting brain remodelling and plasticity for stroke recovery: therapeutic promise and potential pitfalls of clinical translation. Lancet Neurol 2012, 11:369-380.

31 - T. Bliss, R. Guzman, M. Daadi, et al. Cell transplantation therapy for stroke ⌐ Stroke, 38 (2007), pp. 817–826.

32 - Bang OY, Lee JS, Lee PH, Lee G: Autologous mesenchymal stem cell transplantation in stroke patients. AnnNeurol 2005, 57:874-882.

33 - Lee JS, Hong JM, et al. A long-term follow-up study of intravenous autologous mesenchymal stem cell transplantation in patients with ischemic stroke. Stem Cells 2010, 28:1099-1106.

34 - Honmou O, et al Intravenous administration of auto serum-expanded autologous mesenchymal stem cells in stroke. Brain 2011, 134:1790-1807.

35 - Bhasin A, et al: Autologous mesenchymal stem cells in chronic stroke. Cerebrovasc Dis Extra 2011, 1:93-104

36 - riedrich MA, et al: Intra-arterial infusion of autologous bone marrow mononuclear cells in patients with moderate to severe middle cerebral artery acute ischemic stroke. Cell Transplant 2012, 21(Suppl 1):S13-S21.

37 - Hiu, Takeshi, et al. Synaptic Remodelling after Stroke Enhanced by Transplanted Human Neural Stem Cells is Coincident with Functional Recovery Stroke 45.Suppl 1 (2014): A14-A14.

38 - Stone, L. L., W. C. Low, and A. Grande. "Stem Cell Therapies for Ischemic Stroke."Stem Cells and Neurodegenerative Diseases (2014): 142.

39 - Polentes J, et al. Human induced pluripotent stem cells improve stroke outcome and reduce secondary degeneration in the recipient brain. Cell Transplant.2012 Aug 10.

40 - hang DJ, et al. Therapeutic potential of human induced pluripotent stem cells in experimental stroke. Cell Transplant.2012 Oct 3.

41 - teinberg, Gary K., et al. "A Novel Phase 1/2A Study of Intraparenchymal Transplantation of Human Modified Bone Marrow Derived Cells in Patients with Stable Ischemic Stroke." Stroke 45.Suppl 1 (2014): A149-A149.

42 - Kim, Suk J., et al. "Intravenous transplantation of mesenchymal stem cells preconditioned with early phase stroke serum: current evidence and study protocol for a randomized trial." Trials 14.1 (2013): 317.

43 - avitz SI, Dinsmore J, Wu J, Henderson GV, Stieg P, Caplan LR: Neurotransplantation of fetal porcine cells in patients with basal ganglia infarcts: a preliminary safety and feasibility study. Cerebrovasc Dis 2005;20:101-107

44 - Sprigg N, Bath PM, Zhao L, Willmot MR, Gray LJ, Walker MF, Dennis MS, Russell N: Granulocyte-colony-stimulating factor mobilizes bone marrow stem cells in patients with subacute ischemic stroke: the stem cell trial of recovery enhancement after stroke (STEMS) pilot randomized, controlled trial.

45 - avitz SI, Misra V, Kasam M, Juneja H, Cox CS Jr, Alderman S, Aisiku I, Kar S, Gee A, Grotta JC: Intravenous autologous bone marrow mononuclear cells for ischemic stroke. Ann Neurol 2011, 70:59-69.

46 - Friedrich MA, Freitas GR et al: Intra-arterial infusion of autologous bone marrow mononuclear cells in patients with moderate to severe middle cerebral artery acute ischemic stroke. Cell Transplant 2012, 21(Suppl 1):S13-S21.

47 - Lee JS, Hong JM, Moon GJ, Lee PH, Ahn YH, Bang OY: A long-term follow-up study of intravenous autologous mesenchymal stem cell transplantation in patients with ischemic stroke. Stem Cells 2010, 28:1099-1106.

48 - Honmou O, Houkin K, Matsunaga T, Niitsu Y, Ishiai S, Onodera R, Waxman SG, Kocsis JD: Intravenous administration of auto serum-expanded autologous mesenchymal stem cells in stroke. Brain 2011, 134:1790-1807.

49 - Soma Banerjeea, Paul Bentleyb, et al; Intra-Arterial Immuno-selected CD34+ Stem Cells for Acute Ischemic Stroke; Stem Cell Transitional Medicine; Accepted June 16, 2014.

50 - Takahashi K, Yamanaka S et al Induction of pluripotent stem cells from adult human fibroblasts by defined factors. Cell. 2007 Nov 30; 131(5):861-72.

51 - Wang S, Goldman SA et al Human iPSC-derived oligodendrocyte progenitor cells can myelinate and rescue a mouse model of congenital hypomyelination. Cell Stem Cell. 2013 Feb 7; 12(2):252-64.

## CHAPTER 18 CONCEPTS TO CLINIC: Part III

1 - Black, Linda L., et al. "Effect of adipose-derived mesenchymal stem and regenerative cells on lameness in dogs with chronic osteoarthritis of the coxofemoral joints: a randomized, double-blinded, multicenter controlled trial." Veterinary Therapeutics 8.4 (2007): 272.

2 - Sutter, W. "Autologous cell-based therapy for tendon and ligament injuries." Clinical techniques in equine practice 6.3 (2007): 198-208.

3 - Richardson, Lucy E., et al. "Stem cells in veterinary medicine–attempts at regenerating equine tendon after injury." Trends in biotechnology 25.9 (2007): 409-416.

4 - Hani A. Awad, David L. Butler, Gregory P. Boivin, Frost N.L. Smith, PrasannaMalaviya, Barbara Huibregtse, and Arnold I. Caplan. Tissue Engineering. June 1999, 5(3): 267-277

5 - Dan Deng, et al Biomaterials. Oct 2014, Vol. 35: 8801-8809

6 - Abumaree M, Al Jumah M, Pace RA, Kalionis B (2012) Immunosuppressive properties of mesenchymal stem cells. Stem Cell Rev 8:375–392

7 - Philippe Hernigou, et al International Orthopaedics. Sep 2014, Vol. 38: 1811-1818

8 - F. Rayanmarakkar, W. S. Khan, and T. E. Hardingham, "Principles of tissue engineering approaches for tendons, skin, nerves and blood vessels in the hand," in Hand Surgery: Preoperative Expectations, Techniques and Results, R. H. Beckingsworth, Ed., pp. 85–96, Nova Science Publishers, New York, NY, USA, 2009.

9 - E. Oragui, N. Sachinis, N. Hope, and W. S. Khan, "Short communication: tendon regeneration and repair, and the role of mesenchymal stem cells,"

in Mesenchymal Stem Cells, Y. Xiao, Ed., Nova Science Publishers, New York, NY, USA, 2011.

10 - F. Rayanmarakkar, W. S. Khan, A. Malik, and T. E. Hardingham, "Principles of tissue engineering approaches in plastic surgery: tendons and skin," Stem Cell Research, vol. 2, no. 1, pp. 1–10, 2010.

11 - N. A. Siddiqui, J. M. L. Wong, and W. S. Khan, "Stem cells for tendon and ligament tissue engineering and regeneration," Journal of Stem Cells. In press.

12 - J. Donaldson and W. S. Khan, "Functional tissue engineering for rotator cuff tendons," Journal of Stem Cells. 2010;5(4):195-204.

13 - MacLean, S., et al. "Tendon regeneration and repair with stem cells." Stem cells international 2012 (2011).

14 - Koh, Yong-Gon, et al. "Clinical results and second-look arthroscopic findings after treatment with adipose-derived stem cells for knee osteoarthritis." Knee Surgery, Sports Traumatology, Arthroscopy (2013): 1-9.

15 - Mao, Qiang, et al. "The efficacy of targeted intraarterial delivery of concentrated autologous bone marrow containing mononuclear cells in the treatment of osteonecrosis of the femoral head: A five year follow-up study." Bone 57.2 (2013): 509-516.

16 - Jo CH, Lee YG, Shin WH, et al. Intra-articular injection of mesenchymal stem cells for the treatment of osteoarthritis of the knee: A proof-of-concept clinical trial. Stem Cells 2014; 32(5):1254-1266.

17 - Vangsness CT Jr, Farr J 2nd, Boyd J, et al. Adult human mesenchymal stem cells delivered via intra-articular injection to the knee following partial medial meniscectomy: a randomized, double-blind, controlled study. J Bone Joint Surg Am 2014;96(2):90-98

18 - Scott, Ryan T., and Christopher F. Hyer. "Role of Cellular Allograft Containing Mesenchymal Stem Cells in High-risk Foot and Ankle Reconstructions." The Journal of Foot and Ankle Surgery 52.1 (2013): 32-35.

19 - Kim, Yong Sang, et al. "Clinical outcomes of mesenchymal stem cell injection with arthroscopic treatment in older patients with osteochondral lesions of the talus." The American journal of sports medicine 41.5 (2013): 1090-1099.

## CHAPTER 19 CONCEPTS TO CLINIC: Part IV

1 - Alison MR, Islam S, Lim S: Stem cells in liver regeneration, fibrosis and cancer: the good, the bad and the ugly. J Pathol 2009, 217:282-298.

2 - Alison MR, Forbes S et al Hepatic stem cells: from inside and outside the liver? Cell Prolif. 2004 Feb; 37(1):1-21.

3 - Lorenzini, Stefania, et al. "Stem cells for end stage liver disease: how far have we got?." World journal of gastroenterology: WJG 14.29 (2008): 4593.

4 - Dean Yimlamai et al Hippo Pathway Activity Influences Liver Cell Fate; Cell; Volume 157, Issue 6, p1324–1338, 5 June 2014

5 - Seung-Jin Kim, Min Hee Park, Hyo Jung Moon, JinHye Park, Du Young Ko, ByeongmoonJeong. Polypeptide Thermogels As a 3D Culture Scaffold for Hepatogenic Differentiation of Human Tonsil-derived Mesenchymal Stem Cells. ACS Applied Materials & Interfaces, 2014.

6 - Bliss, M. The Discovery of Insulin.25th Anniversary Edition. University of Chicago Press, Chicago; 2007

7 - Fuhlbrigge, Rebecca, and Linda Yip. "Self-Antigen Expression in the Peripheral Immune System: Roles in Self-Tolerance and Type 1 Diabetes Pathogenesis." Current diabetes reports 14.9 (2014): 1-10.

8 - Meier, Juris J., and Riccardo C. Bonadonna."Role of reduced β-cell mass versus impaired β-cell function in the pathogenesis of type 2 diabetes."Diabetes care 36.Supplement 2 (2013): S113-S119.

9 - RicordiC, et al; (2012) From cellular therapies to tissue reprogramming and regenerative strategies in the treatment of diabetes. Regen Med 7:41–48.

10 - ShapiroAM, et al. (2006) International trial of the Edmonton protocol for islet transplantation. N Engl J Med 355:1318–1330.

11 - Domínguez-Bendala J, et al. (2012) Concise review: Mesenchymal stem cells for diabetes. Stem Cells Translational Medicine 1:59–63.

12 - Aguayo-Mazzucato C, et al (2010) Stem cell therapy for type 1 diabetes mellitus. Nat Rev Endocrinol 6:139–148.

13 - Staeva TP, et al. (2013) Recent lessons learned from prevention and recent-onset type 1 diabetes immunotherapy trials. Diabetes 62:9–17.

14 - LysyPA, et al (2012) Concise review: Pancreas regeneration: Recent advances and perspectives. Stem Cells Translational Medicine 1:150–159.

15 - SoriaB, et al. (2000) Insulin-secreting cells derived from embryonic stem cells normalize glycemia in streptozotocin-induced diabetic mice. Diabetes 49:157–162.

16 - Park IH, et al. (2008) Disease-specific induced pluripotent stem cells. Cell 134:877–886

17 - OhmineS, et al. (2012) Reprogrammed keratinocytes from elderly type 2 diabetes patients suppress senescence genes to acquire induced pluripotency. Aging (Albany NY) 4:60–73.

18 - KudvaYCet al. (2012) Transgene-free disease-specific induced pluripotent stem cells from patients with type 1 and type 2 diabetes. Stem Cells Translational Medicine 1:451–461.

19 - MaehrR, et al. (2009) Generation of pluripotent stem cells from patients with type 1 diabetes. ProcNatlAcadSci USA 106:15768–15773.

20 - ThatavaT, et al. (2011) Indolactam V/GLP-1-mediated differentiation of human iPS cells into glucose-responsive insulin-secreting progeny. Gene Ther18:289–293.

21 - Thatava T, et al. (2013) Intrapatient variations in type 1 diabetes-specific iPS cell differentiation into insulin-producing cells. MolTher 21:228–239.

22 - Voltarelli, Júlio C., et al. "Autologous nonmyeloablative hematopoietic stem cell transplantation in newly diagnosed type 1 diabetes mellitus." Jama 297.14 (2007): 1568-1576.

## CHAPTER 20 STEM CELLS AND SPINAL CORD INJURY

1 - Salazar DL, et al Human neural stem cells differentiate and promote locomotor recovery in an early chronic spinal cord injury. 2010 Aug 18; 5(8):e12272

2 - Uchida N, Back SA et al Human neural stem cells induce functional myelination in mice with severe dysmyelination. SciTransl Med. 2012 Oct 10; 4(155):155ra136.

3 - deLázaro, Irene, AçelyaYilmazer, and Kostas Kostarelos. "Induced pluripotent stem (iPS) cells: A new source for cell-based therapeutics?." Journal of Controlled Release 185 (2014): 37-44.

4 - Lu, Paul, Ken Kadoya, and Mark H. Tuszynski."Axonal growth and connectivity from neural stem cell grafts in models of spinal cord injury."Current opinion in neurobiology 27 (2014): 103-109.

5 - Nutt, Samuel. hiPSC-derived Neural Stem/Progenitor Cells in Chronic Cervical Spinal Cord Injury. Diss. 2013.

6 - Ghobrial, G. M., et al. "Promising Advances in Targeted Cellular Based Therapies: Treatment Update in Spinal Cord Injury." J Stem Cell Res Ther 4.170 (2014)

## CHAPTER 21 STEMS CELL AND HIV DISEASE

1 - TakamitsuTerasakiet al Complete disappearance of recurrent hepatocellular carcinoma with peritoneal dissemination and splenic metastasis: A unique clinical course after surgery; Journal of Gastroenterology and Hepatology; Volume 15, Issue 3, pages 327–330, March 2000

2 - Takemura et al Case of spontaneous regression of metastatic lesions of leiomyosarcoma of the esophagus; Diseases of the Esophagus; Volume 12, Issue 4, pages 317–320, December 1999

3 - H. Kappauf et al;:Complete spontaneous remission in a patient with metastatic non-small-cell lung cancer Case report, review of literature, and discussion of possible biological pathways involved; Ann Oncol (1997) 8 (10): 1031-1039.

4 - Evans, Dylan. "Placebo." Mind over matter in modern medicine (2003).

5 - Lokich, Jacob. "Spontaneous regression of metastatic renal cancer: case report and literature review." American journal of clinical oncology 20, no. 4 (1997): 416-418.

6 - Hurwitz, Peter Joel. "Spontaneous regression of metastatic melanoma." Annals of plastic surgery 26, no. 4 (1991): 403-406.

7 - Hütter, Gero, et al. "Long-term control of HIV by CCR5 Delta32/Delta32 stem-cell transplantation." New England Journal of Medicine 360.7 (2009): 692-698.

8 - Galvani, Alison P., and John Novembre. "The evolutionary history of the CCR5 Δ 32 HIV-resistance mutation." Microbes and Infection 7.2 (2005): 302-309.

## CHAPTER 22 DISEASES IN A DISH

1 - Thomas Kahl, et al "Aniline" in Ullmann's Encyclopedia of Industrial Chemistry 2007; John Wiley & Sons: New York

2 - Sheng Ding, PhD – et al . Direct reprogramming of mouse fibroblasts to neural progenitors. ProcNatlAcadSci U S A. 2011 May 10;108(19):7838-43

3 - Rashid ST, et al. Modeling inherited metabolic disorders of the liver using human induced pluripotent stem cells. J Clin Invest. 2010, 120: 3127–3136,

4 - Ring KL, et al. Direct reprogramming of mouse and human fibroblasts into multipotent neural stem cells with a single factor. Cell Stem Cell. 2012, 11:100–109,

5 - Chang DJ, et al. Therapeutic potential of human induced pluripotent stem cells in experimental stroke. Cell Transplant. 2012 Oct 3.

6 - Efe JA, Hilcove S, Kim Jet al. Conversion of mouse fibroblasts into cardiomyocytes using a direct reprogramming strategy. Nature 2012, 485, 593–598

7 - Dimos J, et al K. Induced pluripotent stem cells generated from patients with ALS can be differentiated into motor neurons. Science, 2008, 321:1218–1221, Epub 2008 Jul 31.

8 - Soldner F, et al. Parkinson's disease patient-derived induced pluripotent stem cells free of viral reprogramming factors. Cell. 2009 136:964–977.

9 - WernigM,et al; . Neurons derived from reprogrammed fibroblasts functionally integrate into the fetal brain and improve symptoms of rats with Parkinson's disease. ProcNatlAcadSci U S A. 2008, 105:5856–5861. Epub 2008 Apr 7.

10 - HD iPSC Consortium. Induced pluripotent stem cells from patients with Huntington's disease show CAG-repeat-expansion-associated phenotypes. Cell Stem Cell, 2012, 11:264–278.

11 - Jin Z, Okamoto S, et al. Modeling retinal degeneration using patient-specific induced pluripotent stem cells. PLoS On. 2011 Feb 10;6(2)

12 - Tsuji O, et al. Therapeutic potential of appropriately evaluated safe-induced pluripotent stem cells for spinal cord injury. ProcNatlAcad Sci. USA, 2010, 107:12704–12709, Epub 6 Jul 2010

13 - Jin G, Kim T, et al. Bone tissue engineering of induced pluripotent stem cells cultured with macrochanneled polymer scaffold. J Biomed Mater Res Part A, 10.1002/jbm.a.34425

14 - Hiramatsu K, et al. Generation of hyaline cartilaginous tissue from mouse adult dermal fibroblast culture by defined factors. J Clin Invest. 2011 121: 640–657, Epub: 10 Jan 2011.

15 - Medvedev SP, et al. Human induced pluripotent stem cells derived from fetal neural stem cells successfully undergo directed differentiation into cartilage. Stem Cells Devel. 2011, 20: 1099–1112, Epub 17 Oct 2010.

16 - Efe JA, et a; Conversion of mouse fibroblasts into cardiomyocytes using a direct reprogramming strategy. Nature 2012, 485, 593–598

17 - Qian L, Srivastava D et al. In vivo reprogramming of murine cardiac fibroblasts into induced cardiomyocytes. Nature. 2012, 485:593–598.

18 - Song B, Smink A, et al. The directed differentiation of human iPS cells into kidney podocytes. PLoS ONE 7(9): e46453.

19 - Rashid ST, et al. Modeling inherited metabolic disorders of the liver using human induced pluripotent stem cells. J Clin Invest. 2010, 120: 3127–3136, Epub: 25 Aug 2010.

20 - Jeon K, Lim H, et al. Differentiation and transplantation of functional pancreatic beta cells generated from induced pluripotent stem cells derived from a type 1 diabetes mouse model. Stem Cells and Development. 2012, 21:2642–2655

21 - Szabo E, et al. Direct conversion of human fibroblasts to multilineage blood progenitors. Nature 2010. 468:521–526.

22 - Sheng Ding, PhD – et al . Direct reprogramming of mouse fibroblasts to neural progenitors. ProcNatlAcadSci U S A. 2011 May 10;108(19):7838-43

23 - Izumi et al., 2007;Dissecting the molecular hierarchy for mesendoderm differentiation through a combination of embryonic stem cell culture and RNA interference. StemCells, 25 (2007), pp. 1664–1674.

## CHAPTER 23 STEM CELLS AND AGING

1 - Peck, Douglas T. "Misconceptions and Myths Related to the Fountain of Youth and Juan Ponce de Leon's 1513 Exploration Voyage"

2 - Seluanov, A., et al. Change of the death pathway in senescent human fibroblasts in response to DNA damage is caused by an inability to stabilize 2001. Mol. Cell. Biol. 21, 1552-1564.).

3 -  Kerr JF, Wyllie AH and Currie AR (1972) Apoptosis: a basic biological phenomenon with wide-ranging implications in tissue kinetics. Br J Cancer 26: 239–257

4 -  Wyllie AH (1997) Apoptosis: an overview, Br Med Bull 53: 451-465

5 -  Wright and Hayflick 1975; Muggleton-Harris and Hayflick 1976; Hayflick 1998

6 -  Bodnar AG, Ouellette M, Frolkis M, Holt SE, Chiu CP, Morin GB, Harley CB, Shay JW, Lichtsteiner S and Wright WE (1998) Extension of life-span by introduction of telomerase into normal human cells. Science 279: 349–352

7 -  Fu W, Begley JG, Killen MW, Mattson MP (1999) Anti-apoptotic role of telomerase in pheochromocytoma cells. J BiolChem 274: 7264–7271

8 -  MK Shigenaga, et al; Oxidants, antioxidants, and the degenerative diseases of aging.1993; Proc. Natl. Acad. Sci. pp. 7915–7922.,

9 -  Jovanovic SV, Clements D and MacLeod K (1998) Biomarkers of oxidative stress are significantly elevated in Down syndrome. Free RadicBiol Med 25: 1044–10448

10 -  Orr WC and Sohal RS (1994) Extension of life-span by overexpressionof superoxide dismutase and catalase in Drosophila melanogaster. Science 263: 1128–1130

11 -  Rathbun WB and Holleschau AM (1992) The effects of age on glutathione synthesis enzymes in lenses of Old World simians and prosimians. Curr Eye Res 11: 601–607

12 -  Brown K SIRT3 reverses aging-associated degeneration; Cell Rep. 2013 Feb 21;3(2):319-27.

13 -  Pereira Jet al The in vitro and in vivo effects of a low-molecular-weight fucoidan on the osteogenic capacity of human adipose-derived stromal cells; TissueEng Part A. 2014 Jan;20(1-2):275-84.

14 -  Jensen GS, Hart AN, Zaske LA, et al. (2007) Mobilization of human CD34+ D133+ and CD34+ CD133(-) stem cells in vivo by consumption of an extract from Aphanizomenon flosaquae-related to modulation of CXCR4 expression by an L-selectin ligand. Cardiovasc. Revasc. Med. 8(3): 189-202.

15 -  FraukeNeff et al. Rapamycin extends murine lifespan but has limited effects on aging; J Clin Invest. 2013;123(8):3272–3291

## CHAPTER 24 HEALTHY STEM CELLS LIFESTYLE

1 - Dunac et al. Neurological and functional recovery in human stroke are associated with peripheral blood CD34+ cell mobilization. J Neurol. 2007 Mar;254(3):327-32.

2 - Hill et al. Circulating endothelial progenitor cells, vascular function, and cardiovascular risk. N Engl J Med. 2003 Feb 13;348(7):593-600.

3 - Shintani et al. Mobilization of endothelial progenitor cells in patients with acute myocardial infarction. Circulation 2001; 103:2776-2779.

4 - Leone et al. Usefulness of granulocyte colony-stimulating factor in patients with a large anterior wall acute myocardial infarction to prevent left ventricular remodeling (the rigenera study). Am J Cardiol 2007, 100:397-403.

5 - Lee et al. Reduced circulating angiogenic cells in Alzheimer's disease. Neurology. 2009 May 26;

6 - Lee et al. Decreased number and function of endothelial progenitor cells in patients with migraine. Neurology. 2008 Apr 22;70(17):1510-7.

7 - Esposito et al. Circulating CD34+ KDR+ endothelial progenitor cells correlate with erectile function and endothelial function in overweight men. J Sex Med 2009; 6(1):107-114.

8 - Walter Liszewsk et al Developmental effects of tobacco smoke exposure during human embryonic stem cell differentiation Volume 83, Issue 4, April 2012, Pages 169–178

9 - PrzeglLek et al . Stem cell niches exposed to tobacco smoke. Pub Med. gov 2012;69(10):1063-73.

10 - Deng Y et al Effect of nicotine on chondrogenic differentiation of rat bone marrow mesenchymal stem cells in alginate bead culture. Pub Med. gov Biomed Mater Eng. 2012;22(1-3):81-7

11 - Robert W. Siggins et al Cigarette Smoke Alters the Hematopoietic Stem Cell Niche Med. Sci. 2014, 2(1), 37-50

12 - Kondo et al. Smoking cessation rapidly increases circulating progenitor cells in peripheral blood in chronic smokers. ArteriosclerThromboVasculat Biol. 2004 Aug; 24(8):1442-7.

13 - Otman, W. and Berchtold, N. C, "Exercise: A behavioural intervention to enhance brain health and plasticity," Trends in Neurosciences 25(6) (2002):295-301,

14 - Lee,]., Duan, W., and Mattson, M. P. "Evidence that brain-derived neurotropic factor is required for basal neurogenesis and mediates, in part, the enhancement of neurogenesis by dietary restriction in the hippocampus of adult mice," Journal of Neurochemistry (2002): 1367-1375.

15 - Fung, A., Takase, L., Fornal, C, et al., "Effects of Sleep Deprivation and Recovery Sleep upon Cell Proliferation in Adult Rat Dentate Gyrus," Neuroscience 134(3) (2005): 721-723.

16 - Arasek, M., "Melatonin, human aging, and age-related diseases," Experimental Gerontology 39 (2004): 1723-1729.

17 - Ariznavarreta, C, Castillo, C, Segovia, G., et al. "Growth hormone and aging," Hormones 53(2) (2003): 132-141.

18 - Colao. A., Di Somma, C, Cuocolo,A., et al., "The severity of growth hormone deficiency correlates with the severity of cardiac impairment in 100 adult patients with hypopituitarism: an observation, case-control study," J Clinical Endocrinology and Metabolism 89(12) (2004): 5998-6004.

19 - Jackson KA, Majka SM, Wang H, et al. (2001) Regeneration of ischemic cardiac muscle and vascular endothelium by adult stem cells./ Clin Invest.107(ll):1395-402.

20 - Orlic D, Kajstura J, Chimenti S, et al. (2001) Mobilized bone marrow cells repair the infarcted heart, improving function and survival. Proc. Natl.Acad. Sci. USA 98(18):10344-9.

21 - Lee KD, Kuo TK, Whang-Peng J, et al. (2004) In vitro hepatic differentiation of human mesenchymal stem cells. Hepatology 40:127S-12S4.

22 - Seo MJ, Suh SY, Bae YC, et al. (2005) Differentiation of human adipose stromal cells into hepatic lineage in vitro and in vivo. Biochem. Biophys. Res. Commun. 328, 258-264.

23 - Sordi V, Malosio ML, Marchesi F, et al. (2005) Bone marrow mesenchymal stem cells express a restricted set of functionally active chemokine receptors capable of promoting migration to pancreatic islets. Blood 106,419-427.

24 - Eeberger KL, Dufour JM, Shapiro AM, et al. (2006) Expansion of mesenenchymal stem cells from human pancreatic ductal epithelium. Lab. Invest. 6,141-153.

25 - Camargo FD, Green R, Capetanaki Y, et al. (2003) Single hematopoietic stem cells generate skeletal muscle through myeloid intermediates. Nat lfecf.9(12):1520-7.

26 - Errari b, Lusena-ueangens u, Loieua M, etal.(1998) Muscle regeneration by bone marrow-derived myogenic progenitors. Science 279(5356):1528-9

27 - Krause DS, Theise ND, Collector MI, etal. (2001) Multi-organ, multi-lineage engraftment by a single bone marrow-derived stem cell. Cell 105:369-377.

28 - Pereira RF, Halford KW, O'Hara MD, etal. (1995) Cultured adherent cells from marrow can serve as long-lasting precursor cells for bone, cartilage. and lung in irradiated mice. Proc. Natl. Acad. Sci. USA 92:4857-4861.

29 - Pereira RF, O'Hara MD, Laptev AV, et al. (1998) Marrow stromal cells as a source of progenitor cells for nonhematopoietic tissues in transgenic mice with a phenotype of osteogenesis imperfect. Proc. Natl. Acad. Sci. [7595,1142-1147.

30 - Eglitis MA and Mezey E. (1997) Hematopoietic cells differentiate into both microglia and macroglia in the brains of adult mice. Proc. Natl. Acad. Sci. USA 94, 4080-4085.

31 - Ogle CR, Yachnis AT, Larwell ED, et al. (2004) Bone marrow transdifferentiation in brain after transplantation: a retrospective study. Lancet 363,1432-1437.

32 - Mita M, Adachi Y, Yamada H, et al. (2002) Bone marrow-derived stem cells can differentiate into retinal cells in injured rat retina. Stem Cells 20(4):279-83.

33 - Werner et al. Circulating endothelial progenitor cells and cardiovascular outcome. N Engl j Med 2005; 353(10): 999-1007

34 - Nakagawa, T, Tsuchida, A., Itakura, Y., et al.,. "Brain-derived neurotropic factor regulates glucose metabolism by modulating energy balance in diabetic mice," Diabetes

35 - Feron, E, Burne, T H. J., Brown, J., et al., "Developmental vitamin D3 deficiency alters the adult rat brain," Brain Research Bulletin 65 (2005): 14l-148.'

36 - Stefanie Dimmeleret al HMG-CoA reductase inhibitors (statins) increase endothelial progenitor cells via the PI 3-kinase/Akt pathway 2001) J Clin Invest.;108(3):391–397.

37 - Pereira Jet al The in vitro and in vivo effects of a low-molecular-weight fucoidan on the osteogenic capacity of human adipose-derived stromal cells; TissueEng Part A. 2014 Jan;20(1-2):275-84.

38 - Hamidi S et al fucoidan promotes early step of cardiac differentiation from human embryonic stem cells and long-term maintenance of beating areas; Tissue Eng Part A. 2014 Apr;20(7-8):1285-94.

39 - Shytle DR et al Effects of blue-green algae extracts on the proliferation of human adult stem cells in vitro: a preliminary study; Med SciMonit. 2010 Jan;16(1):BR1-5.

40 - Jensen GS, Hart AN, Zaske LA, et al. (2007) Mobilization of human CD34+ D133+ and CD34+ CD133(-) stem cells in vivo by consumption of an extract from Aphanizomenon flosaquae-related to modulation of CXCR4 expression by an L-selectin ligand. Cardiovasc. Revasc. Med. 8(3): 189-202.

41 - Nina A Mikirova et al Nutraceutical augmentation of circulating endothelial progenitor cells and hematopoietic stem cells in human subjects,1,11 Journal of Translational Medicine' 2010; 8: 34.

## CONCLUSION

1 - Cohen, Cynthia B., and Peter J. Cohen. "International Stem Cell Tourism and the Need for Effective Regulation: Part I: Stem Cell Tourism in Russia and India: Clinical Research, Innovative Treatment, or Unproven Hype?." Kennedy Institute of Ethics Journal 20.1 (2010): 27-49.

2 - Ahmed, Awad M. "History of diabetes mellitus." Saudi medical journal 23.4 (2002): 373-378.

3 - Bliss, Michael. "The history of insulin." Diabetes Care 16.Supplement 3 (1993): 4-7.

4 - Hazlett, Barbara E. "Historical perspective: the discovery of insulin." Clinical diabetes mellitus: a problem-oriented approach (1986): 2-10.

5 - Bessman, Samuel P. "A molecular basis for the mechanism of insulin action." The American journal of medicine 40.5 (1966): 740-749.

6 - McLaren, Anne. "Ethical and social considerations of stem cell research." Nature 414.6859 (2001): 129-131.

7 - McGee, Glenn, and Arthur L. Caplan. "The ethics and politics of small sacrifices in stem cell research." Kennedy Institute of Ethics Journal 9.2 (1999): 151-158.

8 -  Perry, Daniel. "Patients' voices: the powerful sound in the stem cell debate." Science 287.5457 (2000): 1423-1423.

9 -  Sandel, Michael J. The case against perfection. Harvard University Press, 2009.

10 -  Hyun, Insoo. "The bioethics of stem cell research and therapy." The Journal of clinical investigation 120.1 (2010): 71-75.

11 -  Choi HW, Kim JS, Choi S, et al. Neural Stem Cells Differentiated From iPS Cells Spontaneously Regain Pluripotency. Stem Cells 2014;32:2596-2604.

12 -  Plastine, Laura M. "In God we trust: when parents refuse medical treatment for their children based upon their sincere religious beliefs." Seton Hall Const. LJ 3 (1993): 123.

13 -  Cantor, Norman L. "Patient's Decision to Decline Life-Saving Medical Treatment: Bodily Integrity versus the Preservation of Life, A." Rutgers L. Rev. 26 (1972): 228.

14 -  Guichon, Juliet R., et al. "Citizen intervention in a religious ban on in-school HPV vaccine administration in Calgary, Canada." Preventive medicine 57.5 (2013): 409-413.

# Glossary

Acetylcholine: A neurotransmitter released at some synapses in the central and peripheral nervous system as well as at the vertebrate neuromuscular junction.

Adipocyte: A fat cell.

Adult stem cells: Stem cells isolated from tissues after birth, such as bone marrow or epithelium, but also stem cells from the umbilical cord.

Allogeneic transplant: A tissue or organ transplant from an unrelated individual.

Amino acid: An organic molecule that is the building block of proteins.

Angiogenesis: Formation of new blood vessels.

Antibody: A protein made by B cells of the immune system in response to invading antigens.

Antigen: A molecule that stimulates an immune response, leading to the formation of antibodies.

Apoptosis: The process of programmed cell death in case the cell is compromised by infection or other dysfunction.

Autoimmune disease: A disease whereby the immune system reacts against its own tissue, leading to the damage or destruction of specific tissues.

Autologous transplant: A transplant of one's own tissue.

Axon: A long extension of a neuron's cell body that transmits an electrical signal to other neurons.

B cell (B lymphocyte): A type of white blood cell that makes antibodies.

Biopsy: The removal of cells or tissues for detailed examination.

Blastula: An early stage of embryonic development. It consists of a spherical layer of around 128 cells about, 5-8 days after conception.

Blastocyst: The 4-5-day stage of a developing embryo. It consists of the inner cell mass and the trophoblastic.

Carcinoma: Cancer of the epithelial tissue.

Cardiomyocyte: Heart muscle cell.

Cellular membrane: The cellular or cytoplasmic membrane structure that surrounds the cytoplasm. It is the major barrier that separates the inside of the cell from the outside.

Chemokines: "Chemo" means chemical and "kine" means kinetics or movement. Chemokine family are a group of small proteins secreted by cells that affect the mobility or migration of a variety of cells.

Chromosome: One long molecule of DNA that contains a number of genes.

Cytoskeleton: It is the cellular "scaffolding" or "skeleton" within the cytoplasm, responsible for the shape of a cell. It maintains the cell shape, enables cellular motion and plays important roles in intracellular transport, cellular division and cellular migration.

CXCR4: A receptor at the surface of stem cells and other immune cells that has high affinity for a compound called stromal-derived factor-1 (SDF-1).

Dendrite: Short extensions of a nerve cell that receive signals from other neurons.

Differentiation: Is the process by which a stem cell becomes a specialized cell type in a tissue.

Ectoderm: One of three primitive germ layers of a developing embryo. It generates skin, hair, nails, epithelium, sense organs, mouth, and nervous tissue.

Embryogenesis: The development of an embryo from a fertilized egg.

Embryonic stem cell (ES cell): A pluripotent cell derived from the inner cell mass of a mammalian embryo.

Embryonic stem cell line: A culture of ESC, extracted from the blastula that have proliferated in cell culture for several months without differentiating into specific cell types and maintaining their stemness.

Endoderm: One of three primitive germ layers of a developing embryo. It generates the lining of the entire gut, trachea, lungs, bladder, urethra and vagina.

Endothelium: It is the thin layer of cells that line the interior surface of blood vessels. Endothelial cells line the entire circulatory system, from the heart to the smallest capillary.

Enzyme: A protein or RNA that catalyzes a specific chemical reaction.

Epidermis: The epithelial layer of skin that covers the outer surface of the body.

Epithelial cells: Cells that line the cavities and surfaces of structures throughout the body, such as the stomach, intestines, and blood vessels.

Erythrocyte: A red blood cell that contains the oxygen-carrying pigment hemoglobin used to deliver oxygen to cells in the body.

Eukaryote: A cell containing a nucleus and many membrane-bounded organelles. All life-forms, except bacteria and viruses, are eukaryote cells.

Extracellular matrix: Is the tissue that provides structural support to the cells. It makes the connective tissue upon which cells grow and develop into tissues.

Fluorescent microscope: A microscope that is equipped with special filters and a beam splitter for the examination of tissues and cells stained with a fluorescent dye.

Gene: A region of the DNA that holds the code for a specific protein. On division it replicates, so each gene is passed down to all daughter cells.

Genome: All of the genes that belong to a cell or an organism.

Growth factor: A small protein that can stimulate cells to grow and proliferate.

Glial cell: Greek for "glue", glial cells are non-neuronal cells that form the white matter of the brain. They provide support and nutrition to neurons and possibly have other brain functions.

Granulocyte Colony-Stimulating Factor (G-CSF): A glycoprotein produced by various tissues of the body that stimulates the bone marrow to release stem cells into the blood.

Hematopoietic: Greek (haima = blood, and poiesis = to make) It refers to the process of formation of blood cells.

Hemoglobin: An iron-containing protein pigment, located in red blood cells that carry oxygen from the lungs to all tissues throughout the body.

Hepatocyte: liver cell.

Hippocampus: Is a major component of the brain of humans and other mammals. It belongs to the limbic system and plays an important role in emotions and memory.

Histones: Small nuclear proteins, rich in the amino acids, arginine and lysine. They provide the supporting structure for the double helix DNA and chromosomes.

HIV: The human immunodeficiency virus that is responsible for AIDS.

Hormone: A signaling molecule produced and secreted by endocrine glands in one part of the body, and influences tissues in other parts.

Insulin: A polypeptide hormone secreted by beta cells of the pancreas. Its production is regulated by the amount of glucose in the blood.

Interleukin: A small protein hormone, secreted by lymphocytes, to coordinate immune response.

In vitro: Refers to experimentation performed outside of a living organism, for example in a petri dish.

In vivo: Refers to experimentation performed in a living organism, such as a mouse or a human being.

Induced pluripotent stem cell (iPSC): A reprogrammed adult somatic cell that is induced into regaining embryonic properties.

Inner cell mass (ICM). The group of cells that form a lump inside a blastocyst, and gives rise to the embryonic stem cells or a fetus.

Leukocytes: White blood cell.

Leukemia: A cancer of the blood or bone marrow characterized by abnormal proliferation of white blood cells [leukocytes].

Lymphocyte: A type of white blood cell that plays an integral role in the body's immune defense.

Major histocompatibility complex: Genes that code for a large family of cell-surface glycoproteins which bind foreign antigens and present them to T cells use for identification and for induction of an immune response.

Mesoderm: One of the three primitive germ layers of a developing embryo. It generates cartilage, bone, muscle, blood, kidneys, sex organs, and several other tissues.

Metastasis: Spread of cancer cells from the site of the original tumor to other parts of the body.

Mitochondria: Organelle in the cytoplasm, believed to be free-living evolutionary organisms that got incorporated into cells. They produce most of the cell's energy

Monocyte: A type of white blood cell involved in the immune response.

Multipotent: Refers to the ability of a cell to differentiate into a limited number of the body's different cell types.

Mutation: A heritable change in the nucleotide sequence of a gene.

Myelin sheath: Insulation on the axons of neurons. The sheath is produced by oligodendrocytes in the central nervous system and by Schwann cells in the peripheral nervous system.

Myocyte: A muscle cell.

Neurotransmiter: A chemical released by neurons at a synapse, that transmits a signal to another neuron.

Nucleic acid: A macromolecule consisting of a chain of nucleotides. (DNA or RNA)

Nuclear transfer or somatic cell nuclear transfer: The process through which an adult cell is cloned by inserting its nucleus into an egg that has its own nucleus removed.

Oligodendrocyte: A myelinating glia cell of the vertebrate central nervous system.

Osteoblast: Cells that form bones.

Parthenogenesis: A natural form of animal cloning whereby an individual is produced without the fertilization of an egg.

Pathogen: An organism that causes disease.

Phagocytosis: A process whereby cells engulf other cells or organic material by endocytosis.

Placebo: An inert substance that looks the same, and is administered in the same way, as a drug in a clinical trial.

Plasmid: A mini-chromosome, often carrying antibiotic-resistant genes, that occurs naturally among prokaryotes. It is also used as a vector in DNA cloning techniques.

Platelet: A cell fragment derived from megakaryocytes and is involved in blood coagulation.

Plasticity: Ability to permanently change or transform. It also refers to the potential in stem cells to become other cell types.

Pluripotent: Refers to the ability of a cell to differentiate into all types of cells in the body, except for egg and sperm.

Randomized clinical trial: A clinical study in which the participants are randomly assigned to different groups.

Ribosome: A complex of organelles involved in the synthesis of proteins.

Schwann cell: Glia cell that produces myelin in the peripheral nervous system.

Semi-permeable membrane: A membrane that allows certain molecules or ions to pass through it while blocking the passage of other molecules or ions.

Senescence: Refers to the biological processes of a living organism approaching an advanced age. Cellular senescence means the loss of the ability to divide.

Somatic cells: Cells that form the body of an organism, with the exception of stem cells, sperm and ova.

Somatic cell nuclear transfer: An animal cloning technique whereby a somatic cell nucleus is transferred to an enucleated oocyte.

Stem cell: A cell with the ability to develop into a variety of cell types and self-renew itself.

Stromal-Derived factor-1 (SDF-1): Is a compound produced by various tissues that attract stem cells and lymphocytes.

Synapse: A neural communication junction between an axon and a dendrite.

Telomere: The tip at the end of a chromosome, which protects it from fraying and damage.

Teratoma: An encapsulated tumor containing various tissues or organ components, such as liver, lung, hair, teeth, and bones.

Therapeutic cloning: Nuclear transfer with the sole purpose of generating cloned patient-specific stem cells.

Transcription: The copying of a DNA sequence into an RNA molecule

Trophectoderm: The exterior layer of the cells of a blastocyst. It gives rise to the placenta and the membranes.

Unipotent: Refers to the ability of a cell to differentiate only into a single type of cell.

Vector: A virus or plasmid used to carry a DNA fragment into a bacterial or human cell.

Zygote: A diploid cell produced by the fusion of a sperm and egg.

Printed in the United States
By Bookmasters